Linda Madsen

# Translocal Connections of Bioinsecurity

# Zivile Sicherheit

## Schriften zum Fachdialog Sicherheitsforschung

herausgegeben von

Prof. Dr. Dr. h.c. mult. Hans-Jörg Albrecht
Max-Planck-Institut
für ausländisches und internationales Strafrecht, Freiburg

Prof. Dr. Rita Haverkamp
Universität Tübingen

Prof. Dr. Stefan Kaufmann
Institut für Soziologie der Universität Freiburg

Peter Zoche M. A.
Fraunhofer-Institut für System- und Innovationsforschung ISI,
Karlsruhe

Band 14

LIT

Linda Madsen

# Translocal Connections of Bioinsecurity

## Avian Influenza in Turkey and the Becoming of a Global Threat

LIT

The publishing of this book was financed by the Research Council of Norway.

This book is printed on acid-free paper.

**Bibliographic information published by the Deutsche Nationalbibliothek**
The Deutsche Nationalbibliothek lists this publication in the Deutsche Nationalbibliografie; detailed bibliographic data are available on the Internet at http://dnb.d-nb.de.

ISBN 978-3-643-90843-8
Zugl.: Oslo, Univ., Diss., 2014

**A catalogue record for this book is available from the British Library**


Zweigniederlassung Zürich 2016
Klosbachstr. 107
CH-8032 Zürich
Tel. +41 (0) 44-251 75 05
E-Mail: zuerich@lit-verlag.ch http://www.lit-verlag.ch

**Distribution:**

In the UK: Global Book Marketing, e-mail: mo@centralbooks.com
In North America: International Specialized Book Services, e-mail: orders@isbs.com
In Germany: LIT Verlag Fresnostr. 2, D-48159 Münster
Tel. +49 (0) 2 51-620 32 22, Fax +49 (0) 2 51-922 60 99, e-mail: vertrieb@lit-verlag.de

In Austria: Medienlogistik Pichler-ÖBZ, e-mail: mlo@medien-logistik.at
e-books are available at www.litwebshop.de

# Contents

## Preface

This book is the outcome of multiple journeys, as well as spatial, scholarly and social relations, between Turkey, Norway, and later Germany, but it is also strongly influenced by British, Dutch and American connections. The research process entered through a gate constructed with pillars of Beck, Giddens and Lash's sociology of risk. The path would soon take a rather different turn, though. From the very beginning of this project, I was compelled by British geographers' contemporary studies of transboundary animal diseases such as BSE (the so-called mad cow disease), Foot and Mouth Disease, Avian Influenza and, later, Swine Flu. Their approaches fit well with approaches from the field of science and technology studies (STS), the field with which I most strongly identify. The way I have come to understand *biosecurity* and bio*in*security are strongly influenced by these contemporary British studies. Towards the very end of the process of finalizing this book, I have encountered yet another and wider field of security, securitization and insecurity [*unsicherheit*] research, through my recent position as a research fellow at the Centre for Security and Society, at the University of Freiburg. This latter acquaintance has triggered and enabled reflections on the analytical tools I have so far adopted and adapted, and it has made me more conscious and curious about why I let some other approaches go.

I tend to situate the conception of this project to a winter day in early 2006, in the rather unattractive grey steel and concrete staircase at the Faculty of Social Sciences at the University of Oslo. It might sound depressing, but more than ten years later I can still trace the excitement and the motivational rush of inspiration and ideas hatching at that very moment, as I had a chat with Ingunn Moser and she informed me about an upcoming doctoral fellowship at the TIK Centre for Technology, Innovation and Culture. She encouraged me to apply. Eager to do research related to Turkey, a country I knew from previous studies and work, I saw the opportunity to design a research project where I could combine my interest in environmental issues, food security (or, at that time, agricultural risk) and empirical science and technology studies, and where I could study the recent and on-going spread of the poultry disease avian influenza to Turkey.

My project proposal was accepted, and thanks to the tireless support of Ingunn Moser and Kristin Asdal, my motivation persists to this day. This book is a reworked edition of my doctoral thesis. Doubtless, these two highly committed, generous and sharing mentors deserve the honor both for the initiation of this project in the first place and for its completion. Furthermore, I am sincerely grateful to Brita Brenna; your careful reading and detailed comments towards the end of the writing process was invaluable. Any shortcomings are fully mine and mine alone.

The detailed evaluation given and challenging questions raised by Susanne Bauer, Steve Hinchliffe and Göran Sundqvist, who served together in the committee for my doctoral defense, convinced me that this work is of interest and relevance to others; you convinced me about the strengths of my work, and you addressed the shortcomings and weaker points. Some of the latter I have tried to amend.

Fieldwork carried out in Turkey has been essential to this project. Among my contacts in Turkey I would in particular like to thank Prof. Iştar Gösaydin, for helping me with practicalities and for all your useful advice. I am greatly indebted to Rinus Van den Ende: thank you for your hospitality and openness. While our versions of avian influenza in Turkey might differ, my aim has always been to deal with the frictions between these versions in a respectful as well as productive way. I sincerely hope I have succeeded in doing so. It is my ambition and hope that you and your colleagues, who are working hard to prevent and eradicate disease outbreaks, will value this work as a critical but useful contribution to the field.

For reasons of privacy, I address most of my contacts in Turkey by their first name only. I am very grateful to Johanna and Günder: you were key persons for me in that you gave me access to an invaluable network of people in Eastern Turkey. Thank you to Morat for introducing me to relevant people and for guiding me through the eastern provinces. Likewise, thank you to Mansur for helping me to find villages scattered across these provinces, and for introducing me to even more relevant people. I would like to express my sincere gratitude to all of you who welcomed me in your offices, factories, homes, farms and villages where you patiently told me your stories, answered my questions and showed me around. Thank you Nurullah for making me feel at home in Diyarbakır. Among my friends in Istanbul, special thanks goes to Lars Grobe for being the reasonable and steady person who kept me grounded during moments of excitement, and to Lise Berg for motivating me and for triggering excitement once again. Lise acted as my "private virus-alert system" when she notified me about the latest Turkish news, an H5N1 outbreak in Sazköy village by the Black Sea Coast. Thanks to her, I managed to spontaneously travel to this area at the time of the outbreak. This field trip had great influence on the project, and most directly it resulted in all of Chapter 6. I am grateful for the two travel grants given by the The Ryoichi Sasakawa Young Leaders Fellowship Fund (Sylff).

Among my colleagues at the TIK Centre for Technology Innovation and Culture I would especially like to thank Tone Druglitrø and Stefanie Reinert Jenssen for lively discussions and for your social and academic support and cooperation throughout the project. At various stages I have also enjoyed discussions with and feedback from Siv Frøyidis Berg, Beate Elvebakk, Knut Haukelid, Ásdís Jónsdóttir, Christian Lundestad, Sissel Myklebust, Cristine Myravng, Tor-Olav Nævestad, Irene Olaussen, Hilde Reinertsen, Hilde Thygesen, Silje Rem, Lars Risan and Tian Sørhaug.

Natalie Porter, thank you for our exciting discussions and for sharing your experiences from your research of avian influenza in Viet Nam. Thank you for listening patiently to my never-ending discussions about strategy documents. Now these documents are "tamed" in Chapters 4 and 5.

While I often get stressed by the slowness of my writing, my sons, Even ($6^1/_2$) and Henning (4), remind me that I am productive in other ways, at least. Even, thank you for supporting me and for waiting patiently for me to finally finish my *book*. Henning, thank you for reminding me how short the way is from desperate frustration to thrilling excitement. Alex, thank you for taking care of the home and children when I had to spend the weekends and holidays with my laptop rather than with you. Thanks to my parents, Anne and Øivind Madsen, for always being supportive, for your tireless care, for your unquestioning assistance and helpfulness, and for being the best (grand)parents one can possibly dream of!

Last but not least: It is with the greatest thanks to Stefan Kaufmann that this work found its way into the LIT series for *Zivile Sicherheit.* Thank you as well for welcoming me to your research group at the Institute for Sociology and to the Centre for Security and Society in Freiburg. Getting to know Martina F. Biebert, André Biermann, Sabine Blum, Nils Ellebrecht, Sabrina Ellebrecht, Andrea zur Nieden, Elisa Orru, Sebastian Volkmann, and most recently Jens Hälterlein, and being introduced to your heterogeneous sociological approaches to *security*, has triggered awareness and reflections on the advantages of moving beyond the sociology of risk through which I entered. It has made me recognize the influence these approaches have on my own work and on the work of others and it motivates me to go beyond (but not away from!) science and technology studies; it inspires me to continue searching for ways for doing security studies differently – to contribute to different and praxis-oriented studies of security.

# 1. Introduction

What is avian influenza?[1] During this study, I have learned that this question may be answered in many ways. Among them:

**International Organization for Animal Health (OIE):**

> Avian influenza (AI) is a highly contagious viral disease affecting several species of food producing birds (. . . ), as well as pet birds and wild birds. (. . . ) Highly pathogenic avian influenza (HPAI) virus spreads rapidly, may cause serious disease and result in high mortality rates (up to 100% within 48 hours).[2]

**World Health Organisation (WHO):**

> Outbreaks of AI in poultry may raise global public health concerns due to their effect on poultry populations, their potential to cause serious disease in people, and their pandemic potential.[3]

**FAO, OIE and WHO's Global Avian Influenza Strategy (2005):**

> Avian influenza is one of several "emerging transboundary animal diseases (. . . ) [C]ontrol of such trade-limiting diseases is becoming ever more important.[4]

**International field epidemiologist working in Turkey:**

> [In Turkey,] it started in 2005. It was a completely unexpected outbreak in turkeys. . . (smile) – not in *Turkey* but in *turkeys* (laugh) (. . . ) It was clear, it was linked to the wave. . . the wave of [migratory] birds that came from the East, from China, from lake Qinghay (. . . ) Because there. . . suddenly it was (. . . ) a cold wave. (. . . ) the virus must have

1 Throughout the book I may use various terms. Most commonly I write "avian influenza" or "HPAI," depending on what works best in the context and for my argument. Unless otherwise mentioned, this always refers to highly pathogenic avian influenza (HPAI) of the H5N1 strain, HPAI H5N1.

2 OIE Avian Influenza Portal http://www.oie.int/animal-health-in-the-world/web-portal-on-avian-influenza/about-ai/, *read 09.07.2014;* Also in WHO Avian Influenza in animals http://www.euro.who.int/en/health-topics/communicable-diseases/influenza/avian-influenza/history-of-avian-influenza/avian-influenza-in-animals, *read 09.07.2014*

3 http://www.who.int/mediacentre/factsheets/avian_influenza/en/, *read 16.05.2012*

4 FAO, OIE, WHO 2005 May:1 and 2005 Nov.:1, *italics added*

> been *in* some of them, but then... but then, because they were so heavily stressed it was spreading like wild fire (...) it was a very rare event, you know, spreading from wild birds to... That is very rare.[5]

**General manager of one of the five largest poultry-producing companies in Turkey:**

> (...) before the bird flu 60–70% of the chickens were sold in bulk – without any package (...). Now bulk sale is forbidden. The costs of production were like this you know [he holds his hands horizontal above the table, one higher than the other, indicating a big difference in the level of production costs], but now they are equal. That's one way to take out the benefit of this for the consumers but also for the companies ... because it was not fair competition before.[6]

**Neighbour of infected farm in Manyas, north-western Turkey:**

> *Komplot, komplot, komplot*... the European Commission wants to control everything... they want everything to be controlled... There were no bird flu, but the European Union do not want to see free ranging chickens (... ). They want to see that everything is controlled.[7]

Through fieldwork and text work – that is by interviewing a wide range of people who, in various ways, have encountered avian influenza, and by studying documents – avian influenza has become, for me, increasingly complex rather than clearer. Through the answers presented above, avian influenza becomes a "highly contagious viral disease" affecting a wide range of avian species, it is a threat to human health, it is a "trade-limiting disease," it "came from the East," and it is a "*komplot*". These examples show how avian influenza is complex, heterogeneous, and real; real in the form of an obviously lethal disease infecting a poultry flock, or in the form of a conspiracy, materialized by gas containers, burial pits and culling personnel in protective clothes exterminating the backyard poultry stock of entire villages. Moreover, the above answers also demonstrate how avian influenza is a concern to international institutions, to

[5] Interview with international field epidemiologist working for the AI project, *Ankara 29.05.2007* (Interview took place in English)

[6] Interview with Emre Bor, General Manager of Şeker Piliç, *Bandırma 15.05.2007*

[7] Interview with neighbour of outbreak farm in Kızıksa village, Manyas 21.05.2007. Except "*komplot*" this quote is translated from Turkish/ German by me. In this village, many of the men had been working in Germany for years, and our conversations were conducted in a mix of Turkish and German.

industry and individuals, and how it, through the joint efforts of the mentioned world organizations in devising a Global Strategy, is becoming a global issue.

Avian influenza connects the offices of international institutions with individual poultry owners. Moreover, interventions meant to combat avian influenza – and not exclusively the virus itself – affect air travellers and colour the image of the disease in the media. Avian influenza influences, and is influenced by, research priorities. It affects ideas of what is threatened and what is threatening; the virus and its disease stories or aetiology alter ideas of what is good and healthy, and of what is risky or safe. Avian influenza (like other transboundary infectious diseases) disgusts, bores, and annoys. It causes bankruptcy and market opportunities. It is followed by regulatory action, obedience and protest. Hence, this project approaches avian influenza as a matter of biopolitics.[8]

Avian influenza affects and is affected by the way lives are governed; it has implications on, and is implicated by, the ways humans live together – that is what Michel Foucault has addressed as the "biopolitics of the human race".[9] Moreover, avian influenza is just as much about how humans live with non-humans. Again in the words of Foucault, as a matter of biopolitcs, avian influenza is about "control over relations between the human race, or human beings insofar as they are a species insofar as they are living beings, and the environment, the milieu in which they live."[10] Furthermore, avian influenza can be seen in relation to the "subtle, ( . . . ) rational mechanisms" that according to Foucault "become very important in the early nineteenth century" "in order to deal with ( . . . ) phenomena" such as "accidents, infirmities, and various anomalies".[11] The whole apparatus of local, national and transnational institutions, recommendations, procedures, strategies and action plans initiated, fences erected, windows enclosed and medicine and vaccine stockpiled in the name of "progressive[. . . ] control" of avian influenza is continuously materializing how avian influenza is regarded as what Foucault named an anomaly.[12] At the same time, and as the heterogeneous answers above show, control of emerging transboundary animal disease is becoming "ever more important."[13] In this way, avian influenza is simultaneously abnormal *and* normal; dealing

8 Foucault, Michel 2003 [1975–1976]; 2010 [1978–1979]

9 Foucault; Michel 2003: 243

10 Foucault; Michel 2003: 245

11 Foucault; Michel 2003: 244

12 See e.g. the *Global Strategy for progressively controlof highly pathogenic avian influenza.* (FAO, OIE and WHO 2005 May; 2005 Nov)

13 FAO, OIE and WHO 2005 May: 1; 2005 Nov: 1

with anomalies is becoming normal. This alerts us to the importance of studying the biopolitics of normal anomalies such as avian influenza.

While disease and viral infections commonly belong to the domain of biomedicine, the complexities of avian influenza demonstrate that there is more to disease than what can be covered by biomedical approaches alone. This is also a recurring argument and motivation for science and technology studies (STS) of health and disability carried out in the tradition of Foucault and his mentor, Georges Canguilhem[14] Two interrelated points, made by Foucauldian critics of biomedicine and highlighted through disability studies, also serve to emphasise the need for alternative ways of approaching avian influenza. First, these studies show the importance of and they contribute to making space for alternative approaches to issues related to disease, disability and health as a way to work against the increasing dominance of medicine or the medicalization of society. Foucault addressed this "expansion of medicine" and how it is contributing to a particular "disciplinary normalization," as well as how medicine is having regulatory and normative power in the society.[15] The second point, then, is that when medicine contributes to particular normativities where the normal is set as opposed to the pathological, this is pathologizing those who fall outside the norms of the normal. What disability studies demonstrate is how the particular norms and standards set by medicine are not the only alternatives. For example, by taking individual lived experiences into account as measures for (dis)ability, rather than normalizing standards based on population averages, what counts as *able* or not changes substantially.

The zoonotic nature of avian influenza caused by the H5N1 virus, and its potential to cross species barriers and move directly from avian to human species, has made the virus a concern both to human and veterinary medicine. Furthermore, the various implications of avian influenza have triggered market analyses, poultry sector analyses,[16] sociocultural and socioeconomic im-

---

[14] Habraken, Jolanda M, Jeannette Pols, Patrick JE Bindels, Dick L Willems 2008; Moser, Ingunn 2011; 2008 See also e.g. Mol, Annemarie 1998; 2002; Moreira Tiago 2009; Singleton Vicky 2005

[15] Foucault, Michel 2003: 39

[16] Aral Y, Cengis, Yalcin, Yavuz Cevger, Cevat Sipahi, Savaş Sariözkan 2010; Cevger Yavuz, Yilmaz Aral and Cevat Sipahi 2009; Sariözkan Savaş, Cengiz Yalcin and Yalcin, Cengiz 2006; Sayed H. Saghaian, Gökhan Özertan, and Aslıhan D. Spaulding 2008; Sipahi, Cevat, Cengiz Yalcin, Yavuz Cevger, Yilmaz Aral and L. Genc 2011; Yalcin, Cengiz, Cevat Sipahi, Yilmaz Aral, and Yavuz Cevger 2010 The references in this section is a selection, thus not a complete overview, of relevant studies limited to Turkey, but similar studies are certainly carried out on the situation in other countries too.

pact analyses,[17] as well as analyses of public knowledge and compliance with official and/ or scientific advice.[18] These studies and analyses address effects and consequences of avian influenza – of an avian influenza issue already defined by the norms of medicine – and the effects caused by the measures called upon, based on a medicalized understanding of avian influenza. Thus, avian influenza is something that has to be actively dealt with in particular and specific ways. Without contesting the importance of these studies – in fact, several of these serve as valuable resources for this project – this book argues that it is timely to draw attention to *how avian influenza has come to matter in the first place*.[19]

This book takes an approach that is both confrontational and complimentary. By drawing on analytical resources from the field of STS, it takes a processual and relational approach in order to investigate how avian influenza has come to matter. It provides a detailed study of how avian influenza is becoming a heterogeneous and simultaneously local and global matter of concern. Bruno Latour has addressed the distinction between *matters of facts* and *matters of concern*.[20] Put simply, some matters of concern might, through "a long process of negotiation and institutionalization" turn into "indisputable and obvious" matters of fact.[21] Does this mean that matters of fact are more influential and powerful than matters of concern? My argument is that this question should be left open for empirical inquiry and analytical considerations.

Drawing on the analytical approaches of John Law and Annemarie Mol, this book offers insights into how avian influenza is being ordered and enacted through various relations. It details the emergence of a heterogeneous avian influenza issue, and it shows some of the ways in which these multiple avian influenza versions co-exist and move; how they are translated, transported and transformed.[22]

---

17 Geerling, Ellen 2006; Durutan Nedret and Cünyet Okan 2006

18 Sur, Haydar et.al 2007: This reports was informing the *Strategic Communication Framework and Plan for the Prevention and Control of Avian and Pandemic Influenza in Turkey*, carried out by UNICEF on behalf of the Government of Turkey (Unicef Turkey 2006), personal telephone and e-mail communication with Dr Canan Sargin, UNICEF Turkey 09.08.2007(Ankara/Oslo)

19 This argument is drawing on insights from Moser, Ingunn 2008; Fox, Patrick J. 1989; Moreira, Tiago 2009

20 Latour, Bruno 1999; 2004

21 Latour, Bruno 1999: 307

22 See e.g Law, John 1986; 1994; Law, John and John Hassard 2006 [1999]; Mol, Annemarie 2002; Mol, Annemarie and John Law 1994

Finally, this book highlights how the ways in which avian influenza is ordered and enacted contribute to alter what is considered to be safe and unsafe – what is to be regarded bio-secure and bio*in*secure. Thus, in studying how avian influenza has come to matter, I also aim to draw attention to how particular interventions – rather than others – become appropriate, and how such interventions, as means of governance, work to exercise *power over life* – that is, in Foucauldian terms, biopolitics.

## Versions of HPAI H5N1 avian influenza

Thinking of – and with – the heterogenous answers given to my introductory question, on what avian influenza is, one can wonder, like John Law:

> Is it simply that people *believe* different things about reality? Or is it that there are *different realities* being done in different practices? If the first of these positions is right, then we're in the business of beliefs, perspectives and *epistemologies*. If it's the second then we're being backed into issues of *ontology*.[23]

Along with Law, this work is situated within the second position; that of ontology; "in the business of treating reals as *effects of contingent and heterogeneous enactments, performances or sets of relations*."[24] This book does *not* aim to provide *one* answer to the question of what avian influenza *is*. Rather, by studying this emerging transboundary disease, it aims to open up and explore various processes through which avian influenza is *becoming*. It aims to provide space for the multiplicities of highly pathogenic avian influenza (HPAI) of the H5N1 strain; it will study the becoming of various avian influenza versions – some out of many possible.[25]

The ways in which this work aims to study reality – the real – are thus as *multiple*, rather than plural; this book is not about various perspectives, or plurals, which can be valued as more or less good to grasp what avian influenza is about. Neither is it about gathering as many perspectives as possible in order to achieve a total, whole picture. This important distinction is brightly illuminated by Annemarie Mol in her book, *The Body Multiple: Ontology in Medical Practice*.[26] She write about atherosclerosis which, through various practices,

[23] Law, John 2011: 2

[24] *Ibid*

[25] As Marilyn Strathern put it: "The relativizing effect of knowing other perspectives exist gives the observer a constant sense that any one approach is only ever partial, that phenomena could be infinitely multiplied." (2004: xiv)

[26] Mol, Annemarie 2002. For a clear explanation of this difference, see also Mol, Annemarie 2005 [1999]

is enacted in multiple ways; for example through a patient suffering from a painful, discoloured leg in an outpatient clinic, through blood vessels blocked by arteriosclerotic plaque in the operating theatre, and through blood moving through vessels in the Doppler laboratory. Though it is enacted differently in various relations, this is still about one single object, arteriosclerosis; when dealing with *ontologies*, "reality is *done*", or *performed*, and it is "historically, culturally and materially located, then it is also *multiple*" – but "[n]ot plural."[27] For *the* body to work, according to Mol, the various versions have to hold together, to co-exist. So too is avian influenza a single object; the heterogeneous answers to my question above provide a taste of the multiple nature of avian influenza that emerges as it is enacted differently in various relations.

## Ordering

My research questions bring along resources from actor network theory (ANT), the part of STS that pushes the principle of symmetry onto how we deal with human/non-human relations.[28] In line with ANT, this project is not *a priori* dividing human actors and technical and natural objects into active subjects acting on, and passive objects being acted upon, respectively; these divisions, as all other divisions, are not "given in the nature of things" but rather they are "an effect, a product of ordering".[29]

So, this is about *processes and practices*; about (attempts at) making and maintaining order. As Law makes us aware of, order is better seen as verb than as noun; what we are dealing with then, is order*ing*; it takes work and the work never ends.[30] Related to this are the concerns in regards to how orders, labels, categories and classifications are covering up internal variations. For example, Sandra Harding does – with irony, though no less seriously, in the form of a millennium speech – criticize ideas of the end of the 20th century as being "*women's time*"; "the intersectional and multicultural issues alone are enough to make me doubt the usefulness of the [ . . . ] term's falsely unifying energy", she proclaims.[31] However, disadvantageous as they may be, categorization and ordering are unavoidable tools for organizing our minds.[32] Not only keeping

27 Mol, Annemarie 2005: 75

28 See e.g. Akrich, Madeleine 1992; Callon, Michel 1986; Law, John 1986, Latour, Bruno1987; 1988; Star, Susan Leigh 1991; Law, John and John Hassard 1999

29 Law 1994: 10, see also Massey Doreen 2009[2005]; Featherstone, David and Joe Painter (Eds.) 2013

30 Law 1994: 1–2

31 Harding, Sandra 2000:1044. See also e.g. Oudshoorn, Nelly 1999; Star, Susan Leigh 1999

32 See also Lavau, Stephanie 2008: 18

this in mind, but also actively exploring and engaging with variation *within* as well as *between* orders, I aim to turn the drawbacks of orders' unifying effect (orders understood not as absolute and complete, but as a current state of continuous on-going process) into an analytic resource.[33]

Law provides an illuminating image of how and why to do this, by advocating baroque sensibility rather than romantic possibility. "Leibniz is telling us to look for a world of ponds within ponds and gardens within gardens", Law says, and he continues: "instead of looking up we are now looking down (. . . ) at (what is sometimes called) 'detail', rather than up to search for 'the broader picture'. And, as a crucial part of this, we are discovering complexity in that detail."[34] So, what I am searching for is complexity rather than a holistic view. I aim to explore complex and heterogeneous realities – within and among themselves – and how they work together; I will explore the heterogeneities, co-existences, relations and partial connections of avian influenza versions, as they are enacted in different locations, such as for example in global and national strategies for avian influenza preparedness and response, in outbreak reports, villages and offices.[35]

## Re-ordering

By studying and writing about ordering, we are ourselves taking part in ordering and re-ordering. Shapin and Shaffer's writing on Robert Boyle and his air-pump experiments shows how *the modest witness* was produced together with the natural facts that the witnesses were assigned to observe.[36] Through a critical, though appreciative, reading of Shapin and Shaffer's work, Donna Haraway addresses how they contribute to stabilizing and re-stabilizing particular characteristics necessary for the modest witness to possess, in this case "a certain set of masculine virtues".[37] Annemarie Mol makes a similar point: "When critics (. . . ) say over and over again that medicine silences the objects

33 Stephanie Lavau (*Op. cit.)* is doing this in an elegant way as she shows how the multiple realities of Goulburn River is "meandering".

34 Law, John 2002: 19 with references to Deleuze, Gilles 1993 and Kwa, Chunglin 2002

35 On partial connections see Marilyn Strathern (1991); On co-existence see Annemarie Mol (2002), on relations see e.g. Kristin Asdal (2014)

36 Shapin, Steven and Simon Schaffer 1985

37 Asdal, Kristin, Brita Brenna and Ingunn Moser (Eds.) 2007: 26–27; Haraway, Donna 1997. For a similar argument drawing on Haraway, see also Moser (2008: 99) who writes that: "All enactments make a difference, but sometimes they make the same difference, or one that supports other enactments and so contributes to reproduce a pattern rather than diffract and make something new."

of its knowledge, the irrelevance of what patients have to say is restated as many times as a fact".[38] Drawing on Michel Foucault, Mol suggests "noncritical strategies for escaping dominant ways of thinking".[39] "It might be a good way to escape", she says, "from a medicine founded on pathology to wonder whether, in practice, medicine *is* indeed founded on pathology."[40] In a similar vein Ingunn Moser's work on Alzheimer's disease "argue[s] against the 'science-centrism' of parts of STS which privilege science and medicine analytically, and so contribute to the reproduction of their dominance".[41] Thus, when I textualize the becoming of avian influenza in the form of this book, it is with the ambition of continuously reflecting on the ways I contribute to re-order*ing* – rather than to stabilization of *a priori* and taken-for-granted orders – and thus to open up and take into account the avian influenza multiple.

One effective feminist strategy to escape dominant ways of thinking is to draw attention to the excluded; Susan Leigh Star, for example, is sceptical to how ANT is paying too much attention to those that are already powerful, and hence contribute to fortifying these positions and realities.[42] Attending to those that are already included, contributes to re-stabilizing pre-existing power relations. Hence, turning the attention to the excluded, the marginalized and the silenced is what Star recommended we do in order to contribute to making differences. And, who does not want to contribute to making a difference with their research? Taking this apparently immodest position is not necessarily in opposition to Donna Haraway's call for modesty – or an honest kind of modesty.[43] Being a modest witness is not about making oneself invisible, but it is about situating yourself, making your position visible and open for contestation. As pointed out by others, Haraway "argues that scientific knowledge always creates differences. For radical and feminist projects, therefore, this involves participating in the field and helping to make other differences( … )"[44] –

38 Mol, Annemarie 2002: 47

39 *Op.cit.*

40 *Op.cit*

41 Moser Ingunn 2008: 99; See also e.g. Moser, Ingunn 2003

42 See especially Star, Susan Leigh 1991. For a discussion of Star's and others critical contribution to ANT please refer to the introductory chapter in Asdal, Kristin, Brita Brenna and Ingunn Moser (Eds.) 2007, pp. 7–53

43 Haraway, Donna1991; 1997

44 Asdal, Kristin, Brita Brenna and Ingunn Moser (Eds.) 2007:33

that is, to contribute to diffraction.[45] How this can be accomplished – how we can contribute to make a difference – varies.

Kristin Asdal attends to practices through which realities are enacted. This enables her to trace how processes of inclusion and exclusion contribute to establishing certain links, rather than others; hence, certain issues are formed in certain ways, other issues does not come to matter. Regarding her historical study of an aluminium factory in Norway and the adjacent farmland, she finds that "*[n]ot* establishing links between the humans and the animals became a key condition for the making of a new governable space for pollution( . . . )".[46] In this instance "'fluorine' became governable because it was quantified", she claims.[47] Further on, "[t]his quantification helped to create a "political fluorine".[48] The importance given to numbers produced in laboratories in Asdal's text contributes to move laboratory studies *out*, to move them towards empirical studies of politics. Rather than focusing on laboratory work within, it shows how laboratories contribute to enact the outside – through the numbers, relations and realities they produce – and those they do *not* produce.

Moser's work mentioned above contributes to showing how the places of concern of Alzheimer's disease are distributed among a wide range of locations and practices. Studying how the disease is enacted, for example through patients' movements, in advertisement, in parliamentary politics, in a conference on dementia, and in daily care practice, Moser shows that the disease is *also* enacted other places than those that are directly dominated by science and medicine. This involves *inclusion* of more locations, hence inclusion of other processes, objects and subjects. In this way, through inclusion, she avoids restating the position of science and medicine as being exclusive. A further implication of this move to other locations and other practices is that it makes exclusions surface; the ways Alzheimer's disease is made to matter "simultaneously enacts and denies other realities", she writes.[49] Furthermore, in order for some "matters of fact" to emerge and appear stable, differences and tensions "are made absent and invisible, excluded and disarticulated. And this works to unmake them. It makes them less real", Moser writes.[50]

---

45 For an illuminating introduction to Haraway's use of optical metaphors in particular, such as diffraction, but also for a general "manual" to Donna Haraway's work, see Asdal, Kristin, Anne-Jorunn Berg, Brita Brenna, Ingunn Moser and Linda M. Rustad 1998

46 Asdal, Kristin 2007

47 Asdal, Kristin 2007: 309 See also Asdal, Kristin 2011a

48 Asdal, Kristin 2007: 309. Asdal's "political fluorine" is a response to Andrew Barry's (2001) "political chemistry"

49 Moser, Ingunn 2008: 105

50 *Ibid*. See also Law John 2002a; 2003; Law, John and Annemarie Mol 2001

Drawing this point about inclusion and exclusion together, feminist strategies to include the excluded can be seen as a democratizing project, which by avoiding restatements also avoids fortification of already existing power relations. By including, and thus giving the marginalized and excluded a voice, they (or we!) contribute to make a difference, to destabilize power relations and to create other realities.

As I hope is apparent by now, this project is indebted to analytical resources that have emerged, and that are continuously emerging, within the field of feminist science and technology studies. However, by analysing my empirical material in the light of these resources, I have found that my findings complicate or even contradict what is commonly the outcome of such studies. Even though standpoint feminists' claims, that we have to take the position of the weak and suppressed to get the best view, have been complicated by a growing awareness that identities are heterogeneous, changing, open-ended and renegotiated – hence that power(lessness) is situated and relational – the empowering effects of inclusion, and the disempowering effects of exclusions, seem to persist as common assumptions within current feminist technoscience studies. No doubt, this relation can often be found, however it does not mean that it should nor can be taken for granted. In regards to disease events, being kept out, or excluded, might serve valuable and even empowering.

Ordering of avian influenza in Turkey and "globally", as it has been done in global strategies, is more than the result of a process of making absent and present, of exclusions and inclusions. As this project also highlights, it is also about *separation*; it is about enacting versions that are kept apart, and about making some versions mobile and able to travel, and others not, or it is about different versions travelling separate ways. Some versions of avian influenza travel, and contribute to enacting what is becoming "the global avian influenza" issue, while others stay in Turkey and remain domestic matters.[51] It all contributes, in various ways, to enacting avian influenza versions, and to calling for various interventions for "securing life", or "biosecurity interventions".[52] This is a *non-reductionist* story about avian influenza as its spread from Asia to Europe, via Turkey, was reported from 2005 onwards; a story that pays attention to details, that cares about complexities, but the aim of which is not holistic but rather partial. The story(teller) is situated and the approach is diffractive.

---

[51] Asdal, Kristin 2005

[52] Lakoff, Andrew and Stephen Collier (Eds.) 2008; Hinchliffe, Steve and Nick Bingham 2008 b. See also Hinchliffe, Steve, John Allen, Stephanie Lavau, Nick Bingham and Simon Carter 2012

## Mobility

If reality is heterogeneous and a current state of an on-going process of ordering, then the question arises: how do some versions become mobile and others not? Moreover, given that versions are relational, what form do they take when they move from one place to another?

*Mobility* is a central concern within STS. Law and Mol acknowledge the importance of Latour's concept, *immutable mobiles*, for the development of ANT.[53] *Immutable and combinable mobile*s are, according to Latour, facts and technologies that are able to travel long distances, in time and space, and still keep their shape. In order to explain immutable mobiles Latour has used the astronomer Tycho Brahe. Brahe's observations and collections of data on the positions of the planets, his gathering of freshly registered data *and* earlier observations done by other European astronomers which Brahe had access to from older books, are put to work in order for Latour to explain the immutable mobiles: "All these charts, tables and trajectories are conveniently at hand and combinable at will, no matter whether they are twenty centuries old or a day old; each of them brings celestial bodies, billions of tons heavy and hundreds of thousands of miles away to the size of a point on a piece of paper", he writes.[54] What Latour is presenting is thus a network of *immutable* astro scientific facts that are able to keep their shape when they travel between scientists and others interested; hence they were *mobile* in Cartesian, Euclidean or regional space. In this way, again according to Latour, "'the global' was understood as a network for transporting invariant shapes" or immutable mobiles, through regional space.[55] In the case of avian influenza, the standardised forms and the registered data – the so-called Immediate Notification- and Follow-up Reports that are sent to the World Organization for Animal Health (OIE) by responsible authorities in member countries in order to fulfil obligatory notification of disease outbreak – might work as example of such an immutable mobile. Various data considered relevant are registered in forms, in a manner that enables facts concerning unit type, numbers of affected birds, numbers of dead and culled birds, as well as measures taken, to move from outbreak places around the world to the offices of the *World* Organization for Animal Health (OIE).

---

53 Latour, Bruno 1987; Law, John and Annemarie Mol 2001. See also Latour, Bruno 1988; Law, John 1986

54 Latour, Bruno 1987: 227

55 Law, John and Annemarie Mol 2001: 619

Even though facts and artefacts keep their shape, they do not necessarily enact the same realities when they move. And, what about the facts and artefacts that do not move? Or those that do not really keep their shape, those that only partially move, but still work at their new destination? Interested in practices as they (we) often are, those (of us) practising ANT soon realize that, in practice it would be useful to extend the conceptualization of space; in practice, we are dealing with more spatialities; when practising ANT we need more ways to deal with spatiality than what can be grasped as *network space* and *regional space.* Mol and Law have suggested *fluid space* and *fire space*:[56]

> [O]ften enough ideas, facts, information, even technologies, turn out to spread in a manner that is much more *fluid*. It is precisely a lack of rigidity that most helps movement, (... ) If it is successful it is not because the formula is rigid. It is precisely because it can change shape. These, then, are displacements which depend on mutability instead of, or as well as, immutability. Understood in this way globalisation is not about networks but about fluidities. About movements that go more easily if there is less control. About things that take on the shape of their surroundings. That are adaptable.[57]

The "thing" put to work by Law and Mol to illustrate a fluid topology is a bush pump, whose successful working (that is, its ability to pump water of a relatively decent quality), and widespread adoption in many of Zimbabwe's villages, depended on its ability to be repaired and maintained with various bits and pieces at hand. In other words, the bush pump was not dependent on original spare parts; it went on working, despite, or even because if, reparations and adjustments that were changing its shape; the bush pump is a *mutable mobile*.

A quite different "thing" that contributes to demonstrating this topological notion, *fluid space*, is anaemia. Like the bush pump, this one single object, anaemia, may as Mol and Law eloquently show, seem different, and it may be seen differently due to different methods and available technologies, in the Netherlands and in Africa. Anaemia is the same, but different; it too is a *mutable mobile*. Hence, a *fluid topology* is good to think with in studies of anaemia, as in studies of bush pumps and of avian influenza. The latter is the same in China as in Turkey – despite differences. That avian influenza moves between China and Turkey (and potentially any other location) makes it a matter of *globalization*; to paraphrase the so-called global strategy for avian influenza

56 Mol, Annemarie and John Law 1994; Law, John and Annemarie Mol 2001

57 Law, John and Annemarie Mol 2001; 619

control, *all countries are at risk of avian influenza*[58] – still *it*, *the* avian influenza, turns out differently at its different destinations.

Following Law and Mol into *fire space* will not enable us to say more about globalisation; "This spatial metaphor does not explain or even articulate globalisation", they write.[59] Fire is *mutable,* but *immobile*, and they suggest this spatial metaphor "for thinking of the global" and even the universal.

With reference to early STS laboratory studies from the late 1970's, Law and Mol remind us how these studies contributed to shift scholarly attention from epistemology and "the exigencies required of theory" "towards the textures of the practicalities of the laboratory." As they write: "Labelling, marking, repeating, cleaning, numbering, noting, interpreting: these came to be known as the activities which compose science-in-action."[60] In this way science was brought "down to earth"; science is not anymore universal but everywhere; science is inscribed in its objects; "facts are localized". In this way, when matters – avian influenza as any other – are being ordered, earth is getting inscribed in it; hence avian influenza is global; it is becoming a version of the global.

Introducing the topology of fire does not enable us to think about how facts or any other matters move, about regionalization nor globalizations – in those cases we may think with topologies of network or fluid space. By introducing the topology of fire space, Law and Mol encourage us to think behind the global, or as they write, "*to turn universality inside out.*"[61]

To illustrate their point they bring in "a formalism", "an aerodynamic expression" or a "figure" illustrating "'gut response"', "G" – that is what most of us know as turbulence experienced under certain flight conditions.[62] They are showing that what is *present*, "a figure of tolerable G[ut response]", is dependent on what is *absent*:

But that figure depends precisely upon what is *absent* - a sickened and frightened pilot. *Depends upon* that which is absent (so it is present) but (in an additional twist) at the same time depends upon *making* it absent: because there is certainly no room for a pilot and his vomit in the network of relations pencilled on a sheet of paper by an aerodynamicist in a clean office.[63]

---

58 FAO, OIE and WHO 2005 May; 2005 Nov.

59 Law, John and Annemarie Mol 2001: 619

60 Law, John and Annemarie Mol 2001: 609

61 Law, John and Annemarie Mol 2001: 619, *italics in original*

62 Law, John and Annemarie Mol 2001: 618- 619

63 Law, John and Annemarie Mol 2001: 617, *italics in original*

Also, other factors present in the formalist expression are simultaneously both related to and dependent on making matters absent.

> Why does *M*[speed] need to equal or exceed the value of 1? The answer is strategic, and it has to do with Russian military capabilities, real or imagined. (…) [Furthermore,] *W*, weight, leads into the realm of bureaucratic politics (how big to make the aircraft), *S*, size of the wing, to the Russians (the need for short take-off from camouflaged airstrips), and transonic lift slope, $a_t$, not only to high speeds (and so to the Russians) but also aerodynamic wind tunnels (how does a wing behave in practice?)[64]

By being absent, these factors are present as their absence is contributing to this particular formalism. When introducing a topology of *fire space,* Law and Mol "suggested that shape constancy may be understood as a stable pattern of conjoined alterity in which continuity depends upon discontinuity, or presence upon absence, the movement or displacement between here and there."[65]

How might a topology of *fire space* influence how to think of avian influenza? It encourages questions like how avian influenza is being enacted as a global threat in the first place. How is it *becoming* a threat? And, to whom? Moreover, *fire space* provides a context for exploring relational effects of absence/presence, continuity/discontinuity, displacements and "conjoint alterity". This goes well together with the analytical resources already introduced as central resources from feminist technoscience studies in which Law and Mol are deeply involved; how are absent matters contributing to enacting *the* global avian influenza threat?

What *fire space* might add is a specific access point for attending to what is behind the global or the universal. Throughout this book, I will also draw on resources for re-thinking universals developed by the geographer Doreen Massey and the anthropologist Anna Tsing, among others. At the current point, these four topologies of *region-*, *network-*, *fluid-* and *fire space* should provide sufficient analytical equipment to enter the field of avian influenza with a sensitivity to movement and a sharpened attention to how facts, formalisms and universals may be turned inside out in ways that make us consider other versions of reality.

64 Law, John and Annemarie Mol 2001: 617

65 Law, John and Annemarie Mol 2001: 619

## Where to study the local, the global, the global local and/or the local global

This book aims to bring you along on a journey into various sites where highly pathogenic avian influenza is acting and where it is enacted. The particular places considered in this study will be introduced in the next chapter. Here, I will briefly introduce my main motivations for focusing on Turkey in my study of avian influenza.

## Motivation I: Turkey as a melting pot – an opportunity to study pandemics in the making

At the time when I started to plan this project, in 2006, the HPAI (H5N1) avian influenza virus had just recently been detected in Turkey. Turkey was then among the first countries beyond Asia where the HPAI (H5N1) virus was identified, and here several humans were also infected and diagnosed; some had a lethal outcome. The relative sudden geographic spread, combined with detection of several human infections within a short time, resulted in great uncertainty related to how the virus would proceed. These developments drew massive attention; an atmosphere of nervous anticipation was closely coupled with the need for prompt action. With the sudden spread beyond Asia to Turkey, anything could happen. I wanted to grasp the opportunity to follow these developments as they unfolded.

In my preliminary readings on highly pathogenic avian influenza, two characteristics appeared crucial. The potential *pandemic threat* associated with the H5N1 virus that was now circulating was one characteristic that appeared to contribute strongly to the global alarm.[66] With the human incidents, my immediate assumption was that Turkey would represent a strategic place to study both geographic and interspecies viral mobilities.

Secondly, HPAI was primarily referred to as a *poultry disease*. As much attention had so far been paid to the role of markets and trade in the spread of avian influenza in Asia, I assumed that Turkey's position, as a gate, or literally

[66] The "significantly revise[d]" WHO Global influenza preparedness plan of 2005, which replaced the WHO's first pandemic plan published in 1999 and titled *Influenza pandemic plan. The role of WHO and guidelines for national and regional planning,* is one materialized version of what I refer to as global alarm. While these documents were important for my initial reading on avian influenza, neither of these documents receives much attention in this book. Rather, the above-mentioned Global Strategy carried out by FAO, OIE in collaboration with WHO will receive thorough attention, especially in Chapters 4 and 5.

*a bridge*, to Europe, would make it a strategic place to study this *transboundary* disease.[67] I thought the avian influenza spread would make the evergreen metaphor of Turkey as "the bridge between Asia and Europe" greener than ever. The metaphor is pointing at Turkey as a cultural melting pot, and as an important point of passage for travellers, traders, people and goods, moving between the two continents.

Turkey's long journey towards membership in the European Union was another dimension that made this particular country attractive to this project. Already in 1959, Turkey applied for associate membership in the European Economic Community (EEC). Four years later, in 1963, Turkey and the EU signed the so-called "Ankara Agreement". This document primarily marked the path towards a custom union, applicable to all EU member states. For Turkey, it took 32 years to reach the final agreement granting Turkey membership to the EEC. In the meantime, in 1987, Turkey also applied for full membership, and ten years later, in 1997, the country was declared "eligible to become [an] EU member".[68] "[E]ligible", however, did not mean fully prepared and equipped. Before membership-negotiations formally opened in 2005, various projects and reforms were initiated as part of the pre-accession development programs. The aim was to get a wide range of sectors of the Turkish society on the track that would finally lead to fulfilment of the long list of required EU standards. Agricultural and rural development, improvement of veterinary systems, food-control issues, and various phytosanitary measures are examples of some areas particularly relevant for infectious animal diseases that were, and (at the time of writing) still are, to be improved.

At the time when I started this project – and still now, ten years after – the path to EU membership seems long, perhaps even increasingly so. This did not make EU-Turkey interactions less of a motivating factor; focussing on Turkey offered an opportunity to study how the unstable Turkey-EU relations were being influenced when avian influenza was detected in the candidate country, Turkey.[69] I did not intend to make a specific analysis of this relation, and neither

---

67 This assumption was for example based on FAO's Recommendations on the Prevention, Control and Eradication of Highly Pathogenic Avian Influenza (HPAI) in Asia (2004).

68 See e.g. European Commission; Enlargement, Turkey on http://ec.europa.eu/enlargement/countries/detailed-country-information/turkey/index_en.htm

69 One of many examples of growing impatience, or even disbelief in the idea that Turkey will ever join the EU, is a conversation between the famous and Nobel Prize winning Turkish author, Orhan Pamuk, and EU's Commissioner for Enlargement and the European Neighbourhood Policy, Štefan Füle, in October 2012. In a press review, Pamuk had said that "Turkey's EU project 'has fallen apart" Commissioner of Enlargement Füler responded to this, ensuring that "our joint project has not been abandoned" However, he admits "Pamuk's

have I done so. Still, Turkey-EU interactions have crossed my path throughout the work with this book, and have provided an additional *regional* dimension to the "global" UN institutions and the *national* and *local* Turkey.

### Motivation II: The extensive and heterogeneous poultry sector

Turkey has an extensive, expanding and highly diverse poultry sector, something that made it reasonable to assume that this would be a good country for studying various aspects of this poultry disease.[70] Backyard poultry hold, or the practice of keeping *köy tavuğu,* village poultry, is common all over the country. In the case of Turkey, backyard poultry mainly implies a small flock of 6 to 60 birds, primarily hens but ducks and geese may occur as well.[71] This sector is informal. Prior to the avian influenza outbreaks, there was no registration of these birds, and no records indicated the number of backyard poultry in Turkey. These small groups of poultry or individual birds are, however, a very present part of the scenery of any village or neighbourhood. Even in central parts of the city of Istanbul, hens can frequently be seen in backyards and side streets. When the Food and Agriculture Organization of the United Nations (FAO) sent their experts to Turkey in order to evaluate the HPAI situation in 2005/2006, they estimated that this sector counted for 15% – 40% of the total national poultry stock.[72]

Backyard poultry is primarily used for private consumption. You often hear that meat from*köy tavuğu* is regarded as much tastier than the chicken you can buy in the supermarkets. Serving a freshly slaughtered hen from your own flock signals hospitality and good custom, and is a way to honour guests. I had the pleasure of enjoying freshly slaughtered and well-prepared *köy tavuk* at several occasions during my field visits to different areas of the country during my field trips – served with curious smiles and humorous comments that they did not know what else to serve me, or jokes about whether I was nervous about eating these chickens. Eggs from the village hens are used for consumption in the private households. Bartering eggs is also common, but considering the size of these flocks the potential income from marketing eggs

words reflect the mood often felt on both sides ( ... )". http://ec.europa.eu/commission_2010--2014/fule/docs/articles/20121010_turkey_article.pdf (*read 11.07.2014*) *This article was published on the occasion of the publication by the European Commission of its* progress report on Turkey, on 10 October 2012.

70 See. e.g. Akbay, C and I. Boz 2005

71 Geerlings, Ellen 2006 and personal observations throughout all fieldwork.

72 Ivanov, Yanko 2007: 23

is limited.[73] Backyard poultry is easy to hold and involves minimal costs; they scavenge and are fed only occasionally, mainly in the wintertime when other food sources are scarce. Mainly women, children and the elderly take care of these birds, which also have the status as pets. One girl, who had recovered from avian influenza, told me how she, a short time before she turned ill, had brought her chickens inside when they became ill and it was freezing cold outside.[74] She brought them to her bed, where she cared for them. Fortunately, she was the only one to become infected, despite the fact that she lived in a very small house with several siblings and other relatives.

While backyard poultry hold is practiced all over Turkey, industrial poultry production is mainly concentrated in the north-western part of the country. Contrary to what exists for backyard poultry, national statistics provide figures for the industrial poultry sector. According to these numbers, the sector produced five times as much poultry meat in 2005, which was the year when the first HPAI outbreak was detected in October, as in 1990.[75] According to the same statistics, the five largest firms covered 48% of the national broiler production in 2005. Taking into account the next five of the largest firms, these ten together represent 68% of the total national formal white meat or poultry production sector. Due to the avian influenza outbreaks, several medium-scale semi-integrated and integrated firms went bankrupt. Hence, the largest firms came out of the situation with a larger market share; these companies had the capacity and resources to survive the "market shock", to adjust production facilities, and to implement new biosecurity measures. They managed to utilize the potentials for branding that became increasingly important as bulk sale was prohibited and packing became mandatory.[76]

The poultry meat production and the layer production are organized differently. The former is organized in large, vertically integrated firms, which have their own breeder units, hatcheries, feed mills, and often also their own slaughterhouses. The firms use contract farmers to whom they provide day-old chicks or *civciv* (normally around 20.000 birds per batch), feed and pharma-

73 This volume does not aim to provide deep insight into the backyard poultry sector, nor any other sectors of poultry production, but in addition to what I have gleaned from personal observations and interviews Nedret Dürütan and Okan Cüneyt (2006) and Ellen Geerlings (2006) provide useful accounts especially of backyard poultry hold, which prior to the HPAI received minimal research attention.

74 Personal communications with the youngest of surviving avian influenza victims, Van, 11.06.2007

75 Yalcin, Cengiz 2006

76 Personal communication with Director of Finances, Poultry Producing Company, Balıkeşir 15.05.2007; see also e.g. Yalcin, Cengiz 2006.

ceuticals. The contractors feed and care for the chicks until they reach the proper size for broilers, approximately 45 days. Then they are picked up by the company's trucks and brought to the slaughterhouse. In this way, suburban industrial areas where feed mills, slaughterhouses and processing plants are situated, and surrounding villages with contracting farms, are connected. This highlights how "village", a term that is used to categorize the kind of place at which an outbreak is detected (for example in the Immediate Notification and Follow-up Reports forms sent from national authorities to OIE), should not intuitively be assumed to be an isolated, disconnected place. Related to how the poultry production in Turkey is structured, the unit "village" might just as well be an integrated part of the network of larger poultry-producing companies that connects several villages, suburban industrial areas where slaughter, retail, feed mills and company management is situated, and national and international markets.

The layer industry, which produces table eggs, consists of mainly individual medium-scale enterprises, organized in a horizontal integration. Also in this sector, the largest enterprises (farms with more than 50.000 layer hens) represent 65% of the total production.[77] In addition to producing table eggs, this sector is the main provider of "spent hens".[78] Spent layers are hens whose egg production is no longer sufficient due to age or other factors. One of the few studies on backyard poultry in Turkey tells that spent layers are "the major sources of backyard poultry".[79] Another source of spent hens for backyard poultry keepers are those that, also mainly due to age, are discarded from parent stock at large enterprises.

Until the so-called "second wave" of avian influenza, which was characterized by countrywide spread to 53 out of 81 provinces during the winter of 2005/2006, specialized companies collected spent hens from the enterprises.[80] These hens were transported all over the country and sold directly from the trucks or at bazaars. This business was conducted through a large network that both connected poultry all over the country, and that connected the formal and informal poultry sectors, backyards and large-scale commercial coops.[81] During the 2005–2006 outbreaks, spent hen sales got banned, and the Turkish Government offered payment as an incentive for companies to bring these birds to

77 Yalcin, Cengiz 2006

78 See e.g. Durutan, Nedret and Cüneyt Okan 2006; Yalcin, Cengiz 2006.

79 Durutan, Nedret and Cüneyt Okan 2006: point 16; According to Ellen Geerlings (2006) 5–6 million spent hens were annually transported mainly to eastern parts of the country.

80 Geerlings, Ellen 2006

81 Durutan, Nedret and Cüneyt Okan 2006: point 16

specially-equipped slaughterhouses rather than to continue distributing them across the country.[82] Whether the ban was successful has been questioned, and low compensation compared with the market price for these birds is pointed to as a weakness. In relation to disease spread, spent hen sales and live bird markets are of particular relevance because the possibly infected birds involved in this trade might shed and spread virus. Furthermore, highly pathogenic avian influenza has, at least outside Turkey, primarily been associated with large intensive poultry rearing practices such as the places spent hens originate from. Transportation of live poultry, poultry products and eggs are connecting close and remote destinations within and beyond the national borders.

Turkish eggs and poultry products are also exported. Major destinations for Turkish broiler meat are China, Azerbaijan, Hong Kong and Iraq. The latter country also receives 3–4 million Turkish eggs weekly.[83] Shortly before the first detected outbreak of HPAI in Turkey in 2005, six slaughterhouses were certified for export to the European Union market. Five more were in the process of application. This and the subsequent outbreaks brought a temporary, though long-lasting, halt to this market opportunity.[84]

The complex and extensive nature of poultry hold in Turkey offered a good reason to focus on Turkey in my study of avian influenza. Rather surprisingly, though, it is wild birds that have come to occupy large parts of the avian influenza scene in Turkey, and thus also my research.

## Motivation III: Wild birds and migratory flyways

Even from my initial studies of avian influenza carried out in order to write a project proposal, it became apparent that Turkey is not only bridging humans and goods of the two continents Asia and Europe; the country is also working as a transit station for wild birds migrating between Asia and Africa. Maps showing wild bird habitats protected under the Ramsar Convention and wild bird migratory route maps soon appeared in relation to avian influenza outbreaks in Turkey.[85] To what extent migratory routes in particular, and geographical features in general, would be of importance and how such matters

[82] Geerlings 2006:11

[83] Geerlings, Ellen 2006

[84] See e.g. Geerlings, Ellen 2006; Akbay, C. and I. Boz 2006; Yalcin; Cengiz 2006

[85] MARA 2005. The Ramsar Convention is, according to the web site, "The Convention on Wetlands of International Importance ( . . . )[it] is an intergovernmental treaty that provides the framework for national action and international cooperation for the conservation and wise use of wetlands and their resources." (http://www.ramsar.org)

would come to make Turkey a strategic place for studying avian influenza was not known to me when I chose to concentrate on Turkey. I saw it as a potentially relevant and strategic aspect – in addition to the supposedly far more important complex and large poultry sector. What I assumed to be the least important reason for selecting Turkey as site for my study of avian influenza – and also based on what I had so far read about avian influenza in Asia – turned out to be a major matter of attention, though, both of the official disease response in Turkey and of this project.

### Motivation IV: An occasion for returning to Turkey

Concentrating the study on Turkey, I could draw on the advantages of basic Turkish language skills and familiarity with the geography and culture of the country achieved through previous studies and work in Istanbul. This was a valuable experience and highly motivating for my further academic work. In order to navigate efficiently in the Turkish terrain – which includes villages, organisations, academia, as well as public offices – familiarity with and the ability to use the cultural codes and social mechanisms is a prerequisite. My previous experiences were invaluable in this regard. The next chapter offers reflections on some methodological implications related to this.

## Overview of the journey

The next chapter, entitled *Modes of Moving in the Avian Influenza World*, introduces and discusses related methodological approaches and resources that I will work with throughout this book. It also offers an overview and discussion of the multiple field sites of inquiry – that is, primarily sites "out there" in traditional sense, but also "textual sites". The latter will however be more thoroughly introduced in the proceeding chapters where they will be discussed.

Chapter 3 explores the concept *biosecurity*, which, since the turn of this century, has become very central within disease control but which is also widely used within several other fields. Through a performative and relational approach, Chapter 3 analyses how the concept biosecurity is being enacted in recent multidisciplinary academic studies of infectious disease, within the global governance of transboundary diseases, in one particular outbreak situation in Turkey – and in the interface between these sites. This chapter analyses how the concept is allocating significance, substance, meaning and power, as well as how it contributes to making matters significant and how its power contributes to ordering the ways in which to live with pathogens in secure and insecure ways.

Moreover, through these analyses of the concept biosecurity, and my studies of the relations and practices it is part of, I trace how the specific matters of concern tend to be less *securities* than the matters that challenge that which is taken to be secure. Hence, by highlighting the relational nature of biosecurity, this chapter is calling for attention to its rarely mentioned counterpart, addressed here as bio*in*security. Realizing this raises questions about its effect; how does it make a difference to introduce yet another dual concept? How might bio*in*security influence our understanding of biosecurity? The reflections on and expansions of bio(*in*)security posed in this chapter trigger further analytical and empirical moves in the following chapters in ways that can carve out new conceptual tools for studying – thus interfere in – the politics of securing life.

Chapter 4 studies what "the global threat" of avian influenza is becoming when organizations in charge of food and agriculture (FAO) and animal health (OIE) in collaboration with those responsible for human health (WHO) are formulating a common *Global Strategy for Progressive Control of Highly Pathogenic Avian Influenza.*[86] Moreover, how does this "global threat" relate to the national concerns of Turkey when the government is agreeing upon a *National Strategy for Preparedness and Control of Highly Pathogenic Avian Influenza*? Drawing on insights into how texts are making reality – *the realizing effects of textualization* – Chapter 4 studies how these documents are working as textual sites where multiple and heterogeneous versions of avian influenza are being enacted and where they co-exist.[87]

Paying careful attention to the specificities at work in these strategy documents, I trace how avian influenza, in various ways, is being inscribed and enacted as an issue of emerging infectious disease, as an economic issue, as a poultry issue, and as a human health issue.[88] This also involves tracing how

86 FAO, OIE, WHO 2005 Mai; 2005 Nov. These two versions of the Global Strategy are referred to in this volume as the Draft version and Final version respectively. Later global strategies have been made, but as will be explained I concentrate on the two versions published in 2005.

87 On text and reality relations see especially Asdal, Kristin 2007; 2008a; 2008b; 2011a; 2011b; Latour, Bruno 1999, on related argument in regard to e.g. inscription devices, see Latour, Bruno and Steve Woolgar 1979. See also Sundqvist, Göran and Mark Elam 2010; Austin, John L. 1975. On enacting, multiple and heterogeneous reality see Mol Annemarie 2002; 2005 [1999]

88 On *inscription* see Latour, Bruno 1999. On *enacting* see Mol, Annemarie 2002, on *specificities* se e.g. Law, John 2004a

these issues are heterogeneous – how they are enacting different versions – and how these issues and versions thereof co-exist within and between the relational space of these "global" and national documents.[89] Hence, these particular strategy documents also provide sites for studying how avian influenza issues and versions thereof are moving *between* the "global" and the national. Local experiences from outbreaks "on the ground" re-appear in the Global Strategy and text is transferred (apparently by copy/paste) from the Global Strategy to the National Strategy, where the same words reappear in a new, national, context.

According to the Global Strategy, "[a]ll countries in the world are at risk of being infected unexpectedly." Hence, it is a *global problem*. Studying sites such as these strategy documents provide strategic locations for analysing *the becoming of this global problem*. As scholars from various fields have already pointed out, neither universals nor the global are either pre-given or self-evident.[90] In line with this, I suggest that "the global avian influenza problem" should rather be seen as a current outcome of on-going and incomplete localized processes and relations.[91] Hence, in this fourth chapter, I propose that the global may better be seen as relations between local places, which also include the offices of the World Organizations (e.g. WHO, OIE, but also FAO) – the local sites of the global. Suggesting we view the global as part of what might be called *connecting locals*, this chapter invites discussions that might move us beyond vertical "top-down" as well as "bottom-up" or "grass-root" approaches, which still seem to be predominate.[92] Rather, I suggest exploring how the global may better be seen as horizontal or flat networks of flexible relations.

Chapter 5 studies how the avian influenza spread from Asia to Europe is being inscribed in the updated version of the Global Strategy. Bringing forth the attention from previous chapters on text-reality as well as global-local relations, this chapter explicitly brings in *context*. In this way, I seek to contribute to recent efforts to overcome the awkward and ambivalent relation between

89 On *relational space* see Asdal, Kristin 2011b; 2014.

90 See. e.g. Law, John 2002b; Law, John and Annemarie Mol 2008; Massey, Doreen 2004; 2009; Ong, Aihwa 1999; 2005; Tsing, Anna 2005. This argument also goes well together for example with STS laboratory studies, which are showing how "nature" are being turned into scientific facts through the entangled practices of instruments, scientists and inscription devises (See e.g. Latour, Bruno 1987; Latour, Bruno and Steve Woolgar 1979, Knorr-Cetina, Karin 1981).

91 Law, John 1994

92 See e.g. Tsuda Takeyuki, Maria Tapias and Xavier Escandell 2014

context and STS.[93] By making contextualization part of my analyses, I emphasize how the context of the past may be influencing, but not decisive (!) for, current events, and how the ordering of current events are enabling, as well as disabling, issue-formations for the future.[94] Through detailed empirical analysis, I trace how inscribing the events of spread to Europe in the updated version of the Global Strategy contribute to moving avian influenza towards being a wild bird issue. This leads to a discussion on how issues that were, according my analysis in Chapter 4, enacted as *matters of fact* in regards to spread, such as mechanisms related to travel and transportation, are being affected when long-distance spread caused by wild bird migration is coming in as a major *matter of concern* with the text added in order to inscribe the spread in the final version of the Global Strategy.

Having already analysed how inscriptions of outbreaks contribute to enacting avian influenza as a global and national concern in particular strategy documents in Chapter 4 and 5, in Chapter 6 I move on to specific outbreak places in Turkey. In this chapter, I follow the investigations of a series of outbreaks reported during the early months of 2008. Through outbreak investigations, these outbreaks became associated with the Black Sea coast in ways that enabled the conclusion that this was the clearest example to date of the wild bird source of introduction of HPAI. While outbreak situations are messy and complex, outbreak investigations aim to determine what happened; epidemiologists' investigations of outbreaks seek to identify the source of infection and to detect possible ways of spread. This involves ordering work.

Oscillating between reports from outbreak investigations carried out by the national authorities assisted by the above-mentioned AI project and field notes from my own fieldwork at these places, Chapter 6 studies how complex outbreak places are being ordered in a way that is making outbreaks manageable. I analyse how what I call three tools for ordering – referred to as textual inscription of space, mapping, and the copy/paste tool – in various ways contribute to inclusions and exclusions and to making matters absent and present; hence how they contribute to enacting a particular *topology of bio(*in*)security*.[95] This particular topology both limits the possibilities of past events – or what may have caused outbreak – as well as calls for certain interventions, rather than

93 A central contribution is Science, Technology, & Human Values, special issue on Context, Vol. 37, Issue. 4, 2012

94 Asdal, Kristin 2012

95 In doing so, I am drawing on Asdal's "tools of democracy" (2008b) and Law's "moods of ordering" (1994).

others.[96] In extension of this, I show how inscribing outbreak places in such reports involves separation and making some issues mobile, hence enabling them to travel to the international institutions in charge of the global governance of infectious disease, while other versions that are not included in the reports and which is not made mobile and enabled to travel, are, on the other hand, taken care of domestically.[97]

An overall concern of Chapter 6 is to contribute to the efforts of the critics against current global governance – of diseases as well as other matters – who are calling for grounded information as a means to inform, and hence improve, decisions from above.[98] As part of my continuing search throughout this project for alternatives to vertical approaches to local-global relations, this chapter also points at some traps when searching for solutions in the local. By examining the relations between complexity and ordering, this chapter addresses vital implications of allowing inscribed versions of an *emergency* work to inform the *emergent* need for improved preparedness.

Arriving at the final and seventh chapter, I bring along one specific finding of the outbreak investigation studies from the previous chapter, the carcass of a buzzard diagnosed with HPAI H5N1. Along with this deceased (though no less vital) bird – *the* "significant finding" – this final chapter offers a re-view of the book and its major arguments.

---

96 On the relation between past, present and future I am here drawing on Asdal, Kristin 2012 On a suggested move from topography to topology for improving disease prevention and control, see Hinchliffe, Steve, John Allen, Stephanie Lavau, Nick Bingham and Simon Carter 2012

97 Latour, Bruno 1999; Asdal, Kristin 2007; 2011a

98 See e.g. Scoones, Ian (Ed.) 2010; Stirling, Andy C. and Ian Scoones 2009; Scoones and Forester 2008; Leach, Melissa, Ian Scoones and Andrew Sterling 2010.

## 2. Modes of moving in the avian influenza world

*"How did you find your way here? ... How do you know about this place?? ... Who sent you here? Does a firm pay for your trip?" I assure the young farmer and the elderly man accompanying him that I work for a university in Norway, the University of Oslo, and that they pay the costs for my travel. The young farmer takes another look at my card that I had given him some minutes ago when the driver of the* dolmuş, *the public minibus, dropped me off inside their garden (no reason to complain about the service!). Still looking at the card, he nodded his head. The elderly man, who until now had kept himself in the background, stood beside the young farmer and repeated the first questions: how did I hear about this village, and how did I find my way? I told them that I had read about this village on the Internet.* "Internet!", *the elderly man repeated. He continued speaking rapidly to the young man. I could not catch what he was saying, but my impression was that he was amused and excited. I felt the need to elaborate on what I had seen on the Internet.* "Internet'de..." *I caught his attention again. While I was unsure how familiar he was with the Internet, I explained that I had used the Internet to access reports from the Ministry of Agriculture and Rural Affairs and the European Union (EU) about the avian influenza outbreak last winter. Also, on the Internet I had read about the outbreak in online versions of newspapers, the same newspapers as you get in the* bakkal,*the small local shop or kiosk. They both listened to me. This time the elderly man nodded his head. I continued, stretching for my bag, smiling as I told them that I would show them my favourite book. For a second they looked puzzled. I reached for the worn out* Köy Köy Turkiye Yol Atlasi, *Village Village Turkey Road Atlas. The elderly man quickly took it from my hand and began searching through the pages, apparently randomly.* "Sayfa 22," *I said, already familiar with pages 22 and 23 that cover the part of the province where two of the "outbreak villages" from the 2008 outbreaks were situated; one of them was their village, where we were standing right now. The little Black Sea town and administrative centre, where I would be based for the week, was also present on this map.*[1]

Above is a description of a scene from the last of my four field trips to Turkey. It illustrates how I choose places for fieldwork and how I travelled to this location. Like many other places unfamiliar to most people except those

[1] Field notes: 21.10.2008 Konacık village, Karasu District, Sakarya Province

who live there, this village has now had its name inscribed on the global avian influenza maps that are freely accessible, for example on the web pages of OIE.[2] This and other outbreak places, and their "global connections", to borrow Anna Tsing's term, are strategic sites for studying avian influenza.[3] This specific, local place, this village, has become part of something "bigger". But how is a place influenced by, and how is it influencing *the "global threat*" of avian influenza?[4]

Relations between the global and the local and between field and text are among the main analytical matters of concern that will be discussed in this chapter. In this study on avian influenza, I will draw on methodological resources from various fields, which may be characterized as multispecies[5] translocal[6] ethnography, with the aim of investigating multiple sites,[7] embracing the field "out there" in classical ethnographic sense and texts – and the interferences between them.[8] First, I will discuss some general issues related to this before I move on to provide a more specific presentation of my fieldwork. As I will discuss in more detail, I consider texts to be closely connected to the field "out there". Nonetheless, in the presentation of my fieldwork provided in this chapter, I focus mainly on the fieldwork conducted in places "out there", at various places in Turkey. While the most important documents are briefly addressed here, in relation to analytical and methodological discussions, these texts will be introduced in more detail in the respective chapters dealing with them, primarily Chapter 4 and 6.

## Studying avian influenza through its relations

How should one study avian influenza? How does one grasp something that is mobile, fluctuating, indeterminate and invisible? How does one understand

2 OIE Update on Highly Pathogenic Avian Influenza in Animals (Type H5 and H7) ht tp://www.oie.int/animal-health-in-the-world/update-on-avian-influenza/2007, *accessed on 13.07.2014*

3 Tsing, Anna 2005

4 E.g. the Global Strategy is addressing HPAI as a "global threat" (FAO, OIE and WHO 2005 May; 2005 Nov.)

5 Buller, Henry 2013; Haraway, Donna 2008; Hinchliffe, Steve and Sarah Whatmore 2006; Kirksey Eben and Stefan Helmreich 2010; Kohn, Eduardo 2007; Porter, Natalie 2013a; Star, Susan Leigh 1991; Tsing, Anna 2005

6 Tsing, Anna 2005; Tsuda, Takeyuki, Maria Tapias, and Xavier Escandell 2014

7 Marcus; George1995; 2008; Moser, Ingunn 2003; 2005; 2008

8 Asdal, Kristin 2007; 2008a; 2008b; 2011a; 2011b; Latour, Bruno 1999 For a related argument with regards to inscription devices, see Latour, Bruno and Steve Woolgar 1979. See also Sundqvist, Göran and Mark Elam 2010; Austin, John L. 1975.

something that is multiplying or disappearing and that undergoes quick genetic shifts, for example through mutation or re-assortment? My solution is to see avian influenza as something relational; to study how avian influenza is becoming real and how it is being enacted through various relations. Early laboratory studies within Science and Technology Studies (STS) offer analytical resources for studying how the invisible is made visible and "real"; they examine how nature is being turned into scientific facts through the joint efforts of humans, instruments and techniques, and through processes of "heterogeneous engineering".[9]

In this study of the avian influenza virus, I have chosen various places external to, but not disconnected from, laboratories for studying the relations through which avian influenza is being enacted. I have carried out fieldwork in several places where the virus is acting or where it has left its traces – in people's memories or by signs set up by authorities, making the invisible pathogens present and visible.[10] For example, a sign displaying: BURDA KUŞ GRİBİ HASTALIĞI VARDIR, *HERE IS BIRD FLU*, worked as a warning that the HPAI H5N1 virus had been detected; this sign makes it visible that this place has been turned into an outbreak site. And, just such so-called outbreak places are of particular interest throughout this book. In the case of Turkey, places such as gardens, small open chicken coops or villages were turned into outbreak places almost all over the country.

As the excerpt opening this chapter illustrates, I have found my way to these places first by consulting outbreak reports, sent from the Turkish government to the World Organization for Animal Health, where the names of province and district are identified. Subsequently, I either contacted the district officials or found the name of the poultry owners through local newspapers and contacted them directly. Already through the rather short and partial presentations above, multiple sites already appear. One example is one of the many outbreak villages, Konacık. Moreover, national authorities are mentioned; I was keen to meet with district or province authorities, preferably health and veterinary authorities. Furthermore, we get a glimpse of outbreak reports and newspaper articles. A more detailed presentation of the places I have studied and how I chose them will be given later in this chapter. For now, I want to emphasize a more general point: this study is

9 Law, John 1992 For central contributions to laboratory studies see e.g. Latour, Bruno and Steve Woolgar 1979; Traweek, Sharon 1992.

10 Brigitte Nerlich and Nick Wright (2006) point out how measures to fight disease render an otherwise "invisible 'enemy'" visible. I will discuss their contribution in relation to biosecurity in the next chapter.

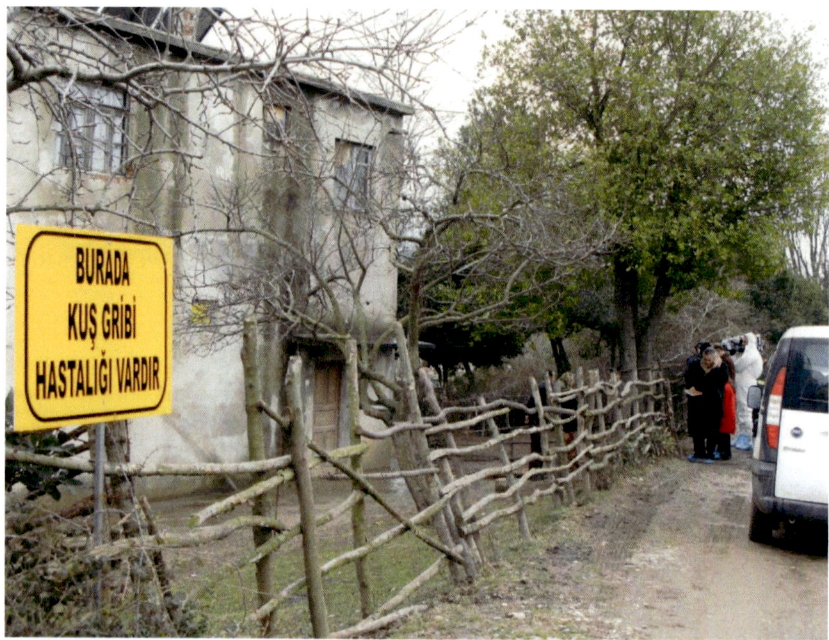


*Picture from field trip to Sazköy Village, Zonguldak Province, 30.01.2008. A sign indicates the presence of "kuş gribi", bird flu. We can see the outbreak house and garden and a film crew interviewing the people living in the house.*

comprised of multi-sited fieldwork through which I take a relational approach to avian influenza.[11] Through this multi-sited fieldwork, I study how avian influenza is enacted at multiple sites "out there" in the field in traditional sense, and "in texts".

## Relating the multiple sites of the field "out there" and "inside text"

By placing quotation marks around the terms "out there" and "in text", I aim to indicate that the borders between such places are unclear; by examining the interferences between the two, it becomes clear that the borders where the field stops and texts begin are not fixed. On the one hand, there is no doubt that the site where the village with the agreed upon name Kızıksa is located exists. On the other hand, this site is dependent on a written confirmation of positive laboratory tests to exist as an outbreak place. To be able to illustrate

[11] Asdal, Kristin 2011a; Marcus, George E. 1995; Moser, Ingunn 2008

this example and mention this particular place at all, I made use of the village name; alternatively, I could have identified the village through its coordinates, but that would only have been another representation.[12] The interdependence between the place "out there" and the positive laboratory result for a place to be enacted as an outbreak place illustrates the interconnectedness of traditional ethnographic sites and texts.

In her work on historical texts, Kristin Asdal illustrates the continuum between text and reality; the reality is textualized and, at the same time, texts realize, she writes; in other words, texts contribute in the making of certain realities.[13] When studying texts related to avian influenza, central questions for this study are: How does this text contribute in making avian influenza real? Drawing on Annemarie Mol's work, I add to this, asking which version(s) of the avian influenza reality are being enacted in certain texts?[14]

Both Donna Haraway and Bruno Latour provide valuable works of inspiration. In his revision of ethnographic methods, George E. Marcus acknowledges their influence on field researchers and their role in stimulating unconventional thinking about such practices. In particular, Marcus mentions that "Haraway's cyborg[15] has been an especially influential construct in stimulating field researchers to think unconventionally about the juxtaposed sites that constitute their objects of study[16]".[17] Thus, for them, as for me, sites are not limited to different settlements, villages or other geographical places. Sites can also be documents, rituals, meetings, tales or pictures. In other words, all kind of places where our topic of interest is practiced represent potential sites of inquiry. Much like the field 'out there', texts may also be seen as places where events unfold; processes taking place in texts are just as interesting as those taking place "out there".

Asdal makes a number of suggestions for how historians can use ethnography. For example, she advocates making use of ethnographic methods in archives, through "redirecting the focus more towards 'how' objects are enacted – and with which effects for the practices in question" instead of being "concerned with exploring archives for the purpose of disclosing 'what' hap-

12 Latour, Bruno 1999

13 Asdal, Kristin 2003; 2008b; 2012; Asdal, Kristin, Kjell Lars Berge, Karen Gammelgaard, Helge Jordheim, Tore Rem, Trygve Riiser-Gundersen og Johan L. Tønnesen 2008

14 Please refer the previous chapter for an introduction on Annemarie Mol's (1999; 2002) work regarding ontology and heterogeneous objects.

15 Haraway Donna 1991

16 Downey, Gary Lee, Joseph Dumit and Sharon Traweek (Eds.) 1995

17 Marcus, George 1995:104

pened".[18] In a similar vein, this project aims to draw on historians' attentiveness to texts. Moreover, I approach texts and the field "out there" symmetrically, in that I study both texts and the field as places where things are happening. I see these as places where processes are taking place; as sites where my object of interest, avian influenza, is being enacted.

Furthermore, drawing on Haraway, Asdal points out that bringing texts or stories together and encouraging them to interact, contributes to producing something more; the outcome of letting two stories work together is something more than the sum of both.[19] I draw on Asdal's work with regards to textualized realities in this study. Though, in addition to allowing various texts written by others to interact, and hence contributing to tease out nuances that may make a difference – that will bring about something new – I also draw on my own field notes and observations. In this context, Tsing's work titled *Friction*, offers a useful guide pertaining to *an ethnography of global connections*.

In her book, Tsing shows how she strives to *grasp the productive moments of misunderstandings*.[20] This illustrates how she makes use of analytical resources: Instead of placing various theoretical views up against each other, she explores their intersections; where some might see conflict, she sees the potential. Tsing writes, "commentators talk right past each other, their intersection could be more productive".[21] It is precisely these *intersections*, *connections*, *encounters* or *confluences* she is dealing with, theoretically but also empirically.[22] Similar to the way Asdal advises us to bring together textualized stories or textualized versions of reality, Tsing proposes the "metaphorical image, *friction*," as a locus for understanding how "heterogeneous and unequal encounters can lead to new arrangements of culture and power."[23] These contributions are informing my work as I study how avian influenza is being enacted as a heterogeneous issue at multiple sites.

## Fluctuating fields, evolving documents and altered versions of the real

The fluctuating, temporal and socio-technical entangled nature of sites can be highlighted when attending to so-called outbreak places. With a positive lab

[18] Asdal, Kristin 2014

[19] *Ibid*

[20] Tsing, Anna 2005: 4

[21] Tsing, Anna 2005: 5

[22] Concepts set here in *italics* are used by Tsing (2005) throughout her book.

[23] Tsing, Anna 2005: 5, *italics added.*

result, a village or an area is turned into an outbreak place. Once the outbreak is controlled and the situation is resolved, the place goes back to "normal" or enters into a "post-outbreak" state. The latter still provides an interesting site for studying an avian influenza outbreak. Indeed, most of the outbreak places I visit were already "post-outbreak places", where outbreaks had already been eradicated by the time I arrived. Although places are declared disease free and outbreaks are officially over, the experience of the outbreak remains present in memories and sighs, and through practices and materialities that have been changed in the name of prevention, disease control or biosecurity. In this way, Serres' philosophy of time as folded or kneaded serves as a good way to think of the co-existence of distant times and present times at (post-)outbreak places.[24]

Within anthropology and geology, there tend to be a working distinction between the social and the natural, or between *bio* or life and *geo* or earth, respectively. The social, bio or life, is seen as dynamic and in process, thus in opposition to nature, geo or earth, which is seen as static and stable. Influential contributions from these fields affect these relations, as well as my work, in many ways. By reading Sarah Whatmore, for example, I have become aware of an early contributor to the field of geography, Carl Sauer, who challenged the previously mentioned bio/geo division. Sauer encouraged geographers to "avoid considering the earth as the scene on which the activity of man (sic) unfolds itself without reflecting that this scene is itself living."[25] Anthropologists' insistence upon traditional, long, "Malinowskian" fieldwork – which, as highlighted by Marcus, are more uncommon than we think[26] – may reflect such an assumption of the field as a stable scene, where both social and cultural processes are unfolding, and where anthropologists may situate themselves over a longer period of time.

Given the fluctuating nature of the "field out there", it is just as interesting to study textualized versions of outbreaks. In a way, outbreak places continue to exist in documents, for example, in outbreak reports. In document format, the outbreak places are made mobile and are able to travel; in their textualized version, outbreaks and outbreak places are travelling and influence what is considered to be "the global threat", as some outbreaks are being inscribed,

24 Serres, Michel 1995. See also Asdal, Kristin 2012

25 Sauer, Carl Ortwin [1925], 1963: 321 quoted in Whatmore, Sarah 2006. According to Whatmore, Sauer is following Vidal de la Blache's argument. See also Massey, Doreen 2005; Featherstone, David and Painter (Eds.) 2013

26 Marcus, George and Judith Okley 2008

for example in the *Global Strategy for the Control of Highly Pathogenic Avian Influenza.*[27]

This example of outbreak places may work to make a convincing argument that places "out there" are unstable and changing. I argue that while a place may continue to exist as an outbreak place in a textualized version, this does not mean that it is fixed; neither the field "out there" nor texts are entirely stable, static or immutable. This is becoming particularly apparent in chapters 4 and 5 of this volume where I analyse texts in detail. For example, the mentioned Global Strategy changes in a physical and material way: it textualizes an "ongoing crisis"[28] and presents itself as an "evolving document".[29] The strategy document states, "the dynamics of the current rapid spread and persistence of HPAI remain unclear."[30] Furthermore, it describes "the changing nature of the AI viruses [and] the role of the complex interactions between the avian influenza virus, the hosts and the changing environment".[31] All this instability and fluidity in the field necessitates flexible documents; documents that can be updated, revised or simply replaced.

Moreover, as will be thoroughly studied throughout this volume, seemingly unchanged texts – words or texts that keep their shape when moving from one place to another – may still be changing. One example is the general concept of "backyard poultry", that moves from Asia where it is referring to particular duck farming practices, via the Global Strategy, to the National Strategy for Turkey where the same concept, "backyard poultry", is working in a new setting, and referring to qualitative different practices of chicken farming. Some vital implications of this particular example will be studied in Chapter 4, but for the sake of methodology, and in relation to working with texts, I put this example into play in order to highlight the unfixed, flexible or mutable nature of texts. As mentioned above, with reference to Asdal, juxtaposing two or more texts will likely produce a sum that is more than the sum of each text

[27] In the previous chapter, I outlined Latour's argument on how observations inscribed in charts and tables are immutable and mobile, how they keep their shape while travelling through time and space. As clarified in Chapter 1, this strategy documents is referred to throughout this volume as the Global Strategy unless it needs to be specified whether I refer to what I simply call the Draft version or the Final version, which is the two editions of this document published in May and November respectively and appear as this in my references: FAO, OIE and WHO 2005 May; 2005 Nov.

[28] FAO, OIE, WHO 2005 May: e.g. 11; FAO, OIE, WHO 2005 Nov: e.g. 15; Ivanov 2007: 42, 72

[29] FAO, OIE, WHO 2005 May: iii; FAO, OIE, WHO 2005 Nov: vii

[30] FAO, OIE, WHO 2005 May: v; FAO, OIE, WHO 2005 Nov: ix

[31] *Op. cit.*

or story combined. To this I will add that reading texts in different settings or contexts may also make it possible to trace how texts are changing and how they influence their contexts; this argument will be discussed further in Chapter 5.[32] Moreover, in Chapter 6, I will trace how an identical text is put to work at several places and how this act of repetition contributes to stabilize a certain reality.

I have now outlined various ways in which texts are flexible or mutable: they may be updated and changed, their meaning or content may change, for example through movement or repetition; and last, but not least, as a matter of methodological self-reflection, texts are both influencing and being influenced by the reader, our reading and re-reading.[33] In this regard, Haraway's re-figuration of the "modest witness" is a powerful reminder.[34] Drawing on the laboratory studies carried out by early STS, and in particular Latour's contributions, Haraway is directing attention toward modern scientists and how they are generally perceived as unbiased producers of neutral facts; that facts are brought forth through pure scientific methods in ways that are objectively mirroring reality.[35] As briefly mentioned above, the contributors to the early STS laboratory studies draw attention to how scientific facts are not simply discovered and unveiled but produced in a heterogeneous network of human efforts, technical and material equipment, circumstances and more. Focussing on how *the scientist* – whose German and Norwegian terms, *der Wissenschaftler* or *vitenskaperen,* can be translated to "the one who brings knowledge into being" or "the creator of knowledge" – are making him- or herself invisible, Haraway emphasises their modesty as false; making one's self invisible and talking on behalf of reality is an *immodest* habit, she claims. Being a modest witness, she suggests, implies not to claim the whole *truth*; it involves being clear and open about your perspectives, and conveying that they are partial and one out of many.[36] Thus, being a modest witness also demands situating yourself in ways that open for critical contestation, but not only that. As modest witnesses we "are not unmarked and neutral, but engaged and localized"; what a modest

32 Asdal, Kristin 2012; Brenna, Brita 2012; Asdal, Kristin and Ingunn Moser 2012

33 The mutual relationship between text and the reader is thoroughly discussed in Asdal, Kristin, Kjell Lars Berge, Karen Gammelgaard, Helge Jordheim, Tore Rem, Trygve Riiser-Gundersen og Johan L. Tønnesen 2008 (*in Norwegian only*)

34 Haraway, Donna 1997

35 For an introduction to STS see e.g. Asdal, Kristin, Brita Brenna and Ingunn Moser (Red.) 2001 in Norwegian or the translated and edited version in English, Asdal, Kristin, Brita Brenna and Ingunn Moser (Eds.) 2007

36 Haraway, Donna 1997; For a user friendly interpretation (in Norwegian only) see Asdal, Kristin, Anne-Jorunn Berg, Brita Brenna, Ingunn Moser and Linda M. Rustad 1998:

witness is doing is "not reflection, but diffraction", that is "creating new and changeable patterns, making a difference".[37]

Bearing this in mind, it is timely to offer some discussion of my own engagement with the material I am working with. Starting with the textualized field, my own influence over the text has been especially apparent in my reading of the mentioned Global Strategy and also of the Turkish National Strategy.[38] By reading these documents repeatedly (and at different times during the project period), I have come to realize that these texts are continuously changing. The realities these texts are enacting are changing with my engagement with the field; the letters, words and pages may be the same, but the stories they tell changes together *with* me, the reader, and *with* other texts, field observations and analytical inputs I have developed since last reading the documents. This is also the case with other documents and texts, but the fact that I have spent extensive time working with these strategy documents makes this process especially evident in relation to these. I began reading these documents at the very beginning of the project; after putting them down for a while, I re-read them once the field trips were completed.

The strategy documents, as well as my strategy for dealing with them, will be discussed in the relevant chapters, 4 and 5. For now, I will only briefly mention how reading with the intention of seeking an answer to the question: "how is avian influenza enacted in these texts?" helped me to "access" the documents; I was able to see through the simple story lines and see how avian influenza was enacted as multiple heterogeneous issues. Through this analytical approach, the documents turned into relational spaces where heterogeneous issues contributed to enacting a "global" and a "national" avian influenza threat. In this way, it also became apparent that within the simple story lines, alternative versions existed that called for other interventions. This makes the documents matters of *biopolitics*. Foucault coined this term in his lectures on governing humans. His focus on humans has triggered critique among scholars otherwise sympathetic to his ideas. Haraway shares her mixed feelings of respect and of being "fooled", telling her readers how she came to realize what she calls a "species chauvinism" in Foucault's work. Recent contribution to the fields of geography, multispecies anthropology and STS have contributed to extend Foucault's term, biopolitics, by using it in studies of governance of non-human populations.[39] Paying attention to how avian influenza is being en-

37 Asdal, Kristin, Brita Brenna and Ingunn Moser (Eds.) 2007: 33; Haraway, Donna 2007

38 Ivanov, Yanko 2007; FAO, OIE and WHO 2005 May; 2005 Nov

39 Haraway, Donna 2008: 60. See Asdal, Kristin 2008a; Asdal Kristin, Christian Borch and Ingunn Moser 2008; Hinchliffe, Steve and Nick Bingham 2008; Hinchliffe, Steve and

acted in documents and in other places is important with respect to biopolitics, as the way avian influenza is enacted, or as Foucault argues, the way knowledge is derived, contributes to "defin[ing] its power's field of intervention".[40] How, biopolitics, biosecurity and not least bio*in*securities of avian influenza is enacted is the major concern of the following chapter.

A final reflection, for now, on how my own engagement influences the material I am studying, relates to how my reading of the documents and my fieldwork observations are influencing each other. Moving between texts and the field, it becomes evident how the fieldwork influences the ways I am reading documents, for example the reports from outbreak investigations. On the other hand, my reading about the outbreak in these reports in advance of my field trip to outbreak places, influences the manner in which I attend and engage in the field. This will be discussed further in Chapter 6, where I pay particular attention to outbreak investigations and the epidemiologists' ordering of complex and messy outbreak places as inscribed in the outbreak investigation reports.

This also illustrates Haraway's point that "[e]very story in a 'field' alters the status of all the others. (...) Altering the structure of a field is [however] quite different from replacing false versions with true versions".[41] By opening up the grand narratives and taking excluded or alternative versions onto account, we can contribute to a more complex, however never complete, image of reality; to use Strathern's illuminating illustration, we may see a whole image, but not an image of a whole.[42]

## Mapping terrain and exploring partial connections[43]

Referring to Zygmunt Bauman, Law reminds us that "orders are never complete."[44] Orders, Law says, "are more or less precarious and partial accomplishments that may be overturned. They are, in short, better seen as verbs rather than nouns."[45] Hence, he suggests we talk about order*ing*. Furthermore, Law rejects "the dream, or the nightmare, of modernity", that is "the idea that

---

Stephanie Lavau 2013; Hinchliffe, Steve and Sarah Whatmore 2006; Kirksey, Eben and Stephan Helmreich 2010; Lemke, Thomas 2014; Lowe, Celia 2010; Porter, Natalie 2013a

40 Foucault, Michel 2003 [1976]: 245

41 Haraway, Donna 1986: 81

42 Strathern, Marilyn 2004

43 The notion "mapping terrain" is taken from George Marcus (1995) and "partial connections" from Marilyn Strathern (2004).

44 Law, John 1994: 1

45 Law John 1994: 1–2

there is a *single* order".[46] Rather, he calls for acceptance of order*ing*, as "plural and incomplete processes of social ordering."[47] Finally, he rejects the notion he just mentioned, "social ordering" because "what we call the social is *materially heterogeneous*: talk, bodies, texts, machines, architectures, all of these are implicated in and perform the 'social'."[48] Hence, he suggest a more suitable notion, that is "sociotechnical ordering".[49]

What do I draw from this? Drawing on both Asdal and Law, I will argue that texts are *tools for sociotechnical ordering*. Furthermore, and in line with both Marcus and Tsing, I move between multiple texts and 'multiple places out there' as I explore how avian influenza is ordered. Avian influenza outbreaks are complex events and establishing clarity demands ordering work. What Marcus refers to as "mapping terrain" has strong parallels to what Law refers to as ordering reality. Similar to Marcus' rejection of holistic representation, Law denies a single order; there might well be one reality but this is a heterogenous reality. The title of Mol's influential book, *Body Multiple,* also emphasises this; *the* body is one, but it comes in multiple versions. For the body to go on living, the different versions must hold together and co-exist.

Drawing on Haraway's cyborg, which is neither human nor a machine, Marilyn Strathern offers an illuminating illustration on this topic.[50] Strathern argues she is "using the connected, non-comparable parts of a cyborg in a double way". She is speaking from the perspective of an anthropologist and a feminist, and the cyborg-metaphor emphasises her point that "neither position" offers "an encompassing context or inclusive perspective. Rather, each exists as a localized, embodied vision." To illustrate her point, Strathern argues that being "an anthropologist is to use feminist scholarship as a resource for or as an *extension* of anthropological insights (... )".[51] The other way in which she is making use of the metaphor of "the unconnected, non-comparable parts of a cyborg" is with "the notion of a machine connected to an organism in the way a tool extends the body suggests a connection between entities based on the fact that *each realizes capacities for the other: each make the other work*."[52] I take Stratherns reworking of Haraway's cyborg as a motivation to engage analytical resources from various fields into my investigation of avian influenza; some of

46 *Op. cit*
47 *Op. cit.*
48 *Op. cit.*
49 *Op. cit.*
50 Strathern, Marilyn [1991] 2004, referred to in Mol, Annemarie 2002: 78–82
51 Strathern Marilyn 2004: 40, *italics added*
52 Strathern Marilyn 2004: 39

these fields have are already mentioned in this chapter, for instance anthropology, geography, history, philosophy, feminist technoscience and STS. This metaphor may also work as a tool to study interrelated objects, such as avian influenza and "the global", which may be seen as set of heterogeneous relations.

## "Where would one locate the global in order to study it?"

This question, raised and answered by Tsing, invites for useful methodological considerations. As previously mentioned, avian influenza is considered a *global threat*. This book will focus on both local and national matters of concern in Turkey, and global concerns as they are being enacted through the mentioned Global Strategy. I seek to examine the relationship between the local and the global, and how to undertake ethnographic research on such seemingly different units.

I draw on the works of Tsing and Strathern to answer the research questions, particularly with regards to notions of the global. They suggest that the global is not an all-embracing, encompassing whole but rather a network of local connections where the global is being enacted in the nodes where two or more versions of the local connect. This brings the global "down to earth" and is reminiscent of Law and Mol's argument, introduced in the previous chapter, where they emphasise how the earth is inscribed in any object, including the global.[53] Again, I can make use of the Global Strategy for demonstrating this point: rather than seeing the Global Strategy as a place where the "global nature" of avian influenza is reflected or mirrored, this document represents one place where avian influenza is being enacted as a global issue. Hence, studying the global is about locating connections and examining the "nodes" where the global is being enacted; the Global Strategy is one site where avian influenza becomes a global issue.

This way of thinking of the global may better be dealt with as what I suggest to address as *connecting locals*. It may also serve as a way of re-thinking what still appears to be a dominant assumption: that the "global" influences, affects, or is translated, consumed, incorporated, re-interpreted or responded to locally, without considering whether or how local forces contribute to the production and reproduction of the "global".

Even though some are pointing out that what is often referred to as "global" is actually rather transnational or translocal, little attention is paid to how these

53 Law John and Annemarie Mol 2001: 619

more or less global objects or matters arise in the first place. Among the exceptions here are Doreen Massey and Tsing, who both warn against what commonly is taken as pre-given and universal.[54] In this volume, I aim to study how what is being referred to as "the global threat" of avian influenza comes into being. In order to study the global, Tsing's solution is to look at "zones of awkward engagement", "global interconnections", and "'worldly encounters", as well as to examine the "awkward, unequal, unstable and creative qualities of interconnection across difference"; Tsing refers to the latter as "'friction"'.[55] Hence, I will examine how local events, in particular specific outbreaks of avian influenza, are interpreted, translated, transported and made to circulate, and how they together with other local outbreaks contribute in enacting what is *becoming* the global avian influenza issue.

If the global should be seen as an encompassing whole it would not have been an easy task to define where to study the other "unit" of this project: Turkey. The country is smaller than the global, but still an overwhelming mass of land, humans, poultry, languages, connections and complexities. Therefore, drawing on Tsing's question used as the heading of this section, the title and the matters of reflection for the next section are as follows:

## Where would one locate the Turkish in order to study it?

I will now present some of the places I have chosen to study the Turkish, or more precisely, the becoming of the heterogeneous Turkish avian influenza issue. After circulating in Asia for almost a decade, the first outbreaks of high pathogenic H5N1 avian influenza virus were first detected in Europe, or more precisely in Romania and Turkey, in October 2005.[56] This was only four months before I initiated this project. As I was sitting in Istanbul the following winter, writing my project proposal, new outbreaks were reported almost daily. I accessed outbreak reports published on OIE's web pages, EU statements and information from the responsible ministries, namely the Ministry of Health (MOH), the Ministry of Agriculture and Rural Affairs (MARA) and the Ministry of Environment and Forestry (MEF). I noticed that the ministries' web pages, which had all been under construction three years earlier while I was working on my master's thesis, had become operational. The websites pro-

54 Massey, Doreen 2003; 2009; Tsing Anna 2005. See also Featherstone, David and Joe Painter (Eds.) 2013; Hecht, Gabrielle 2012; Ong, Aihwa 1999; Ong, Aihwa and Stephen J. Collier (Eds.) 2005

55 Tsing, Anna 2005:4

56 See FAO, OIE and WHO 2005 May: Appendix 2; 2005 Nov: Appendix 2

vided information, documents and reports. Substantial information was available in English, especially concerning avian influenza, which was apparently considered more of an international issue rather than a domestic one. Moreover, at this point, my Turkish skills had also improved. This was a crucial advantage when moving around in the virtual and textual space as well as in physical, geographical space.

### Orientation phase: Reading texts at my desk(s)

In practice, the fieldwork had already begun in Oslo shortly after my project proposal was accepted, and before my first field trip to Turkey. Or perhaps it started a year earlier, when I wrote the project proposal in Istanbul. My research began by examining the Global Strategy mentioned above, published by the Food and Agriculture Organization (FAO) and the World Organisation for Animal Health (OIE) in collaboration with the World Health Organization (WHO). National strategies formulated by the Turkish Ministry of Agriculture and Rural Affairs (MARA) and the Ministry of Health (MOH) were also among the first sites for studying the virus. How was avian influenza acting in these documents? What was it doing? Where and how did it travel? These seemed to be central questions in public debate as the virus suddenly, though not unexpectedly, made a move to Europe and soon to Africa. I became aware of the attention these questions were receiving. Avian influenza in poultry caused by the H5 and the H7 subtypes is a so-called notifiable disease, meaning that, "for the purpose of international trade" OIE member-states are obliged to report any detected incident of infection of these virus subtypes in poultry.[57] I studied the Immediate Notification reports and the following Follow-Up Reports sent by the Turkish national authorities to the OIE. Furthermore, I studied other documents, scientific articles and newspaper articles, especially those covering the outbreaks in Turkey. Through studying these documents and texts, I became aware of the different situations and places where the bird flu virus had been detected, and where it was expected to appear in the future.

### Studying multiple sites in Turkey

In May 2007, I travelled to Turkey for my first field trip. I began the two-month trip in Istanbul (number 1 on the map below) where I spent a week

[57] OIE Terrestrial Codex, Chapter 10.4 Avian influenza Art.10.4.1, http://web.oie.int/eng/normes/mcode/en_chapitre_1.10.4.pdf, *read 09.05.2014*

undertaking practical preparations. Prior to departure, I made a list of people and organizations that I wished to meet. During my first days in Turkey, I tried to reach these people. I encountered a range of problems: The phone numbers didn't work, the switch boards of organisations refused to put me through to the relevant staff member, the line was lost, or when I decided to visit some of the organizations the addresses did not exist or the building was occupied by a totally different entity. On one occasion, I was offered tea in a place I suspected was a brothel, while the service minded portiere took his time trying to determine if anyone had heard of the environmental organization that, according to my notes, was registered to this address.

In light of recent news in Norway about extensive fraud related to the membership numbers of several Norwegian nongovernmental organisations who were seeking to increase their government funding, my immediate assumption was this organization did not really exist, rather, it only had a name and a bank account number. Later I leaned that several street names had been changed and as a result, locating an address could be rather confusing in that part of the city. Rather than an incident of fraud, this proved how vital the relation between street name, as a form of text, and place or location, is.

The turning point happened rather unexpectedly. In a telephone shop, I offered to help two Dutch women who could not speak Turkish. When their problem was solved we had a small talk and the women invited me to join them for bird watching together a local ornithologist. This chance encounter led to the discovery of various ornithological and environmental organizations; it also led me straight to a EU-funded project group, which had begun assisting the Turkish Government in handling the avian influenza only two months earlier, in March 2007. The project, called the Technical Assistance to Avian Influenza Preparedness and Response Project in Turkey (AI project), will appear frequently throughout this book. The twenty-three month project was a central part of the government's avian flu management, and it was very valuable for me to meet this team during the early stages of my work.

The second breakthrough also happened during the first days of my trip, when a former colleague of mine in Turkey offered to introduce me to a relative, a director of a hospital in eastern Turkey. His presence, and in some cases the mere mention of his name and title, gave me access to provincial health and veterinary authorities, recovered bird flu victims, treating doctors, and professors at the university hospital. Each person he introduced me to put me in contact with three, four or five other relevant people. The snowball effect was overwhelming.

## Strategic choices or go with the flow?

From time to time, I had the feeling I was surfing endless waves of strange coincidences and good fortune. During these moments, I would ask myself: What was my original plan? Where did I want to go? Who did I want to meet? Why? How does my field report fit to my initial plans? Am I accomplishing what I planned?

As previously mentioned, my plan was relatively open. However, less than a week after my arrival, the days filled up quickly on account of being introduced and referred to so many different people. The anthropologist Helena Wulff planned short "yo-yo field trips" by making arrangements and appointments in advance; however, she also made sure that she had time for unexpected opportunities that often appear during field visits.[58] Even though I had few appointments in advance, I still had a clear idea of what I wanted to achieve, and opportunities certainly did appear.

During the first year of the HPAI H5N1 outbreaks in Turkey, which occurred in the winter of 2005/2006, a total of 230 outbreaks were detected in 53 of Turkey's 81 provinces.[59] As it was impossible for me to visit all the outbreak places, I had to decide which ones I would visit. I decided to visit Manyas province, the area where the first outbreak was identified (number 2 on the map below). I also visited one of the largest poultry producers in the country and the outbreak village where local farmers were growing broiler chickens for this and other large poultry manufacturer in the area. I continued my trip to Ankara (number 3 on the map below), the capital and administrative centre where I met representatives working for the national authorities working to combat bird flu, including staff from the AI project.

The final destination, according to my plans to reach the eastern city of Doğubeyazit (number 6 on the map above) located in Ağri province, as this was the only place in Turkey where humans that were reportedly infected with the virus had died.[60] As it was practical to pass by Diyarbakir (number 4 on the map above) on the way to Ağri province, I made plans to spend some time there, as several outbreaks had been detected in this area along with the nearby towns of Batman and Silvan both in 2006 and 2007.[61] I was keen to meet with representatives from the local veterinary and health authorities and to visit affected villages. I also stopped in Van (number 5 on the map above),

58 Wulff, Helena 2002; Fangen, Katrine 2005

59 See Geerlings, Ellen 2006

60 WHO 2006

61 These outbreaks will be mentioned in Chapter 6.

which was also on the way towards Ağri province. Through a mixture of good fortune and connections, I was able to meet a wide variety of people, ranging from ornithologists to recovered bird flu victims, treating doctors, (previous) owners of backyard poultry and municipality staff. Finally, I reached my final destination, Doğubeyazıt (number 6 on the map above), which is situated close to the Iranian border.

While I had a considerable amount of time to visit several different places and interview a broad range of people during my first field trip, the following three trips were shorter and their details were planned in advance. By the time I embarked on my later field trips, I was more experienced and it was necessary to make choices about what information was most pertinent to follow up on. In Steve Hinchliffe's study on the British Government's inquiry on Bovine Spongiform Encephalpoathy (BSE), commonly known as mad cow disease, the author explains how he handled the vast range of archival materials by selecting particular episodes or issues; this approach resembles what Tsing calls "ethnographic moments".[62] Hinchliffe maintains that the materials were not selected randomly. Rather, "they had emerged from a long process of following controversies, arguments and debates through the empirical materials that were available".[63] One of the topics or issues that soon stood out as a matter of interest in the Turkish avian influenza response work, and which also appeared to be a matter of international debate, was the role of wild birds in spreading the avian influenza.[64] I therefore saw it as a good opportunity to examine this aspect further when I was allowed to take part in a wild bird catching technique course in Samsun organised by the AI project (number 7 on the map above).

Approximately four months later, in January 2008, I travelled to the Black Sea village, Sazköy, only one week after the outbreaks were detected. This was the closest I got a "face to face" encounter with the virus, and to witness the scene of an outbreak. Field trips normally need to be planned some time in advance. At the same time, and as discussed above, being considered an outbreak place is a temporary condition. A village or an area is turned into an outbreak place and a centre of events after suspicious signs have been detected. Further, positive laboratory results stabilize the status of a site as an outbreak place, but at the same time it intensifies the response activities striving to eradicate

62 Hinchliffe, Steve 2001; Tsing, Anna 2005

63 Hinchliffe, Steve 2001: 187

64 The focus on wild birds was apparent during the analysis of the first outbreak of HPAI in Turkey, where the MARA report (2005) and my interviews with the representative from the AI project illustrate the plurality of answers to the question*: what is avian influenza?* (Interview with international field epidemiologist working for the AI project, *Ankara 29.05.2007*).

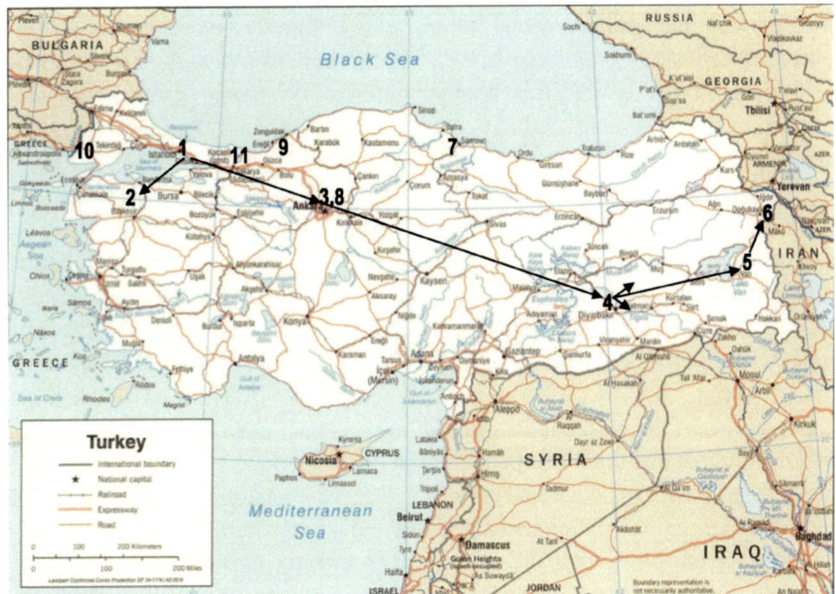


*Map with numbers displaying sites for fieldwork in Turkey. Reference of original map: U.S. Central Intelligence Agency 2006. The map has been modified.*

*1)* ***Istanbul****: starting point; spring 2007*

*2)* ***Manyas****: first detected outbreak, most important area for commercial production; spring 2007.*

*3)* ***Ankara****: capital and administrative center; spring 2007.*

*4)* ***Diyarbakır*** *and* ***Batman****: several outbreaks were detected in these provinces both in 2006 and 2007; spring 2007.*

*5)* ***Van****: location of the University Hospital where people infected with bird flu were treated and place of residence of* **two** *recovered bird flu victims; spring 2007.*

*6)* ***Dogubeyazıt*** *and* ***Agrı****: the tows where people died during the bird flu outbreaks; spring 2007.*

*7)* ***Samsun****: wild bird catching technique course organised by MARA and the AI project; autumn 2007.*

*8)* ***Ankara****: February 2008.*

*9)* ***Sazköy****,* ***Zonguldak*** *province: First of seven detected outbreaks in 2008; February 2008*

*10)* ***Esetçe village, Ipsala district, Edirne Province****; among the seven detected 2008 outbreaks; autumn 2008*

*11)* ***Yenicam and Konacık villages, Sakariya province****; among the seven detected outbreaks in 2008 and Turkey's second most important area for commercial production; autumn 2008.*

the outbreak and further altering the place. It is therefore a rare but useful opportunity to visit an outbreak place during the time of outbreak. As I returned to Norway after this field trip, another outbreak was soon reported followed by further five outbreaks. All these came to be associated with the Black Sea shoreline.

Half a year later, I was finally able to return for the final field trip. I travelled to Turkey to partake in an avian influenza simulation exercise. The simulation exercise was postponed at the last moment, and I instead used the opportunity to carry out fieldtrips to the majority of the so-called Black Sea outbreak places I had yet to visit. Even though half a year had passed since the outbreaks, the memories were fresh in people's minds. As always, their stories, their rejections and my observations of the places contributed to enacting several versions of the outbreak in addition to versions I could trace in the reports and documents that had been published in the immediate aftermath of the outbreaks, and which I had studied carefully. The new versions that emerged from my field trips made vital nuances within the documents more visible. This so-called wave of outbreaks is the matter of concern in Chapter 6 of this book.

As I will discuss in Chapter 6, outbreak places "out there" as well as outbreak investigation reports, which may be seen as textualized versions of these outbreak places, provide strategic sites in a double sense. They are strategic sites for epidemiological investigations aiming to study the introduction and spread of avian influenza; hence they are also strategic sites for me to study how this knowledge production or ordering work contributes in enacting avian influenza. In this regard it is crucial to consider what STS laboratory studies have alerted us to. Similar to in laboratories, events or "pure reality" cannot simply be extracted from outbreak places.[65] Drawing on this literature, I enter outbreak places presuming that, through the practices of outbreak investigation, "the natural" and "the social" are both *realizing capacities for the other*; the use of Strathern's formulation captures the productivity of relations well.[66] A vital implication of this approach is that outbreak places and the epidemiological tools and actors through which they are ordered, are seen as heterogeneous, complex and intertwined.[67]

[65] Haraway, Donna 1997; Knorr-Cetina, Karin 1991; Latour and Woolgar 1979; Shapin and Schaffer 1985; Traweek, Sharon 1992

[66] Strathern, Marilyn 2004: 39

[67] Haraway Donna 1997; 2007

## Methodological implications

In the following section, I will discuss some methodological implications based on practical fieldwork experiences. First, I will say something about having access to, and the chance to talk with, people. Then, I will present some reflections on being what I call a *strange stranger*, a position that is probably familiar for most ethnographers. Whether you are doing fieldwork in "your own culture" or among "exotic tribes people", you are a stranger because the social relationship involves you studying "them". That is strange, and worth reflecting on.

### Getting access, getting around and getting into talk

In a multi-sited fieldwork situation, getting access and making contact with people are something one has to deal with over and over again. Each new place I visited had different experiences with avian influenza, with varying levels of severity. In some areas children had died from the disease. In other places, the social consequences were significant. In some areas, a farmer or family were given the responsibility of culling all poultry in the village after the virus was detected among birds belonging to his household and he had notified the authorities. It is impossible to know what to expect at each location. Almost without exception, I was met with hospitality and openness. When visiting local health and veterinary authorities or other professionals, they often put me directly in contact with a relevant person from the next place I was scheduled to visit; the "snowball" was rolling.

During my first field trip, I found it especially surprising how openly people from the local authorities spoke about the chaotic situations during the countrywide outbreaks in the winter of 2005/2006, and about how ill-prepared they had been. What I heard was in sharp contrast to the descriptions in the detailed action plan published by MARA four years earlier.[68] Once the outbreaks were over and Turkey had regained its status as an avian influenza free country, the general evaluation was that the outbreak situation had been handled successfully. To determine whether this relaxed atmosphere was caused by the positive outcome of the official evaluation is outside the scope of this project. However, whatever the reasons were, the openness was a great resource for my work.

In addition to civil servants, medical doctors and veterinarians, I was keen to meet with owners of the poultry in which the virus had been detected. This

[68] MARA 2001

was surprisingly easy in most cases. Either representatives from the local veterinary or health authorities took me directly to their house, or I found their names in local or national online newspapers and contacted them directly.

Making a good first impression was crucial during my short field visits, as there was no chance to correct a bad start. When introducing myself and outlining the purpose of my visit, I made sure to mention I was undertaking bird flu research. On rare occasions this made people unwilling to talk. At some places, people refuted that any outbreak of avian influenza had taken place. They could explained that "they" or "the people from Ankara" had come and taken all the chickens, geese, and ducks and so on, but they still rejected avian influenza. The people referred to the incident as "nothing",[69] a "mistake", [70] or a "conspiracy".[71] Other times they invited me for tea in the garden or inside their house and asked how they could help me. From time to time, they apologised: "You've come way too late. There is no bird flu here now!?"[72]

Many of the backyard poultry owners I met with started the conversation by saying they did not know anything about the situation, and that they were sorry that they could not help me. A woman told me that her husband was not at home, so unfortunately he could not help me.[73] I asked who took care of the chickens and she answered, nodding towards the elderly woman behind her: "My mother used to take care of them, but now we don't have any chickens anymore. (…) we didn't take any new ones after [they were culled during the bird flu outbreak]"[74]. It was not at all a problem that her husband was not home; I preferred to talk with her mother, the poultryless poultry holder.

At some places where outbreaks had taken place, people were less willing to talk. It was just as interesting to observe these places and their surroundings, as it was to hear their stories. I did not spend much time in the few places where people were unwilling to talk; I spent only a few hours in some areas. Regardless of the length of my stay, I always made observations that added something to the texts I was studying. In that way, visiting these outbreak places has indeed contributed to adding details to the bird flu picture – a picture that will

69 Field notes: 21. 10.2008 Konacık village, Karasu District, Sakarya Province, *my translation from Turkish*

70 *Op. cit.*

71 Field notes: 15.05.2007 Kızıksa village, Manyas District, Balıkesir Province, my *translation from Turkish.*

72 Field notes: 21. 10.2008 Konacık village, Karasu District, Sakarya Province, *my translation from Turkish.*

73 Field trip 15.10.2008, Esetçe village, Ipsala District, Edirne Province

74 Field trip 15.10.2008, Esetçe village, Ipsala District, Edirne Province my translations

never be complete. This might well be "a whole image but not an image of a whole", as Strathern writes, again with reference to Haraway's cyborg.[75]

The fieldwork took place mainly in small villages, neighbourhoods or office buildings. It was not possible for me to hang around in any of these places and observe until I got an impression of the place and its people, until I felt comfortable, or until I meet someone "naturally". I was also *observed*, and if I did not immediately introduce myself, people would become sceptical and suspicious.

## Being a strange stranger

During my field trips, I have come to realize that I am a stranger in at least two ways, and strange in several ways. First, I am a stranger in Turkey; I am obviously not Turkish and I am certainly not from any of the places I visit. Furthermore, I am also strange because I travel a long way to ask strange questions. It is strange that I speak Turkish, and when I do speak the language, it is with a strange accent. In addition, I am strange because I am travelling alone, and the fact that I am a woman makes this even stranger.

Second, I am an academic stranger; it is strange that I study avian influenza even though I am neither a veterinarian nor a medical doctor – my background is in the social sciences. Moreover, I did not expect it would make things any clearer if I announced that I hold an M.A. in science and technology studies and that I am undertaking interdisciplinary research. Furthermore, my position would not have been clarified by mentioning that social anthropology was the major of my B.A., as anthropology is not a predominate field in Turkey. During my previous fieldwork in Turkey, carried out as part of my master's thesis, I interviewed managers of textile factories. During that time, I tried to avoid the confusion of interdisciplinary studies by introducing my work as environmental studies. However, when using the Turkish term for environment, *çevre*, I had to work hard to convince my informants that it was not the economic environment of trade in textile products, but rather environmental impacts and pollution involved in the production process, that I was interested in researching. In my study of avian influenza, I ended up mentioning *sosyoloji*. This subject, sociology, seemed familiar to those I met, and even though my formal training in sociology is rather limited, this word worked to create a familiar ground where people seemed comfortable sharing their experiences and their expertise on avian influenza. It positioned us on a ground where people I met

75 Strathern, Marilyn 2004: 36

patiently and openly told me how their poultry became ill, how they themselves became ill, and how their condition worsened despite taking medication initially prescribed against pneumonia.[76] In addition, veterinarians explained how they had contributed to the culling of the poultry;[77] a medical doctor conveyed how they had been able to immediately determine from the x-rays that their patients were not suffering from pneumonia – but certainly from another ailment;[78] and others discussed how avian influenza had affected their family business and re-positioned their firm within the commercial poultry sector.[79]

As soon as my informants realized that my interest in the issue was sincere, and that I actually was studying avian influenza, they made great efforts to inform me, to teach me, and to do what they could to provide me with a considerable amount of information. They made good efforts to make my travel all the way from Norway to their office or village worthwhile. Sharon Traweek, the anthropologist of science, has famously detailed her experiences of being a woman anthropologist undertaking research among male nuclear physicists.[80] Traweek's story is about disrespect, harassment and chauvinism because of her gender as well as her discipline. Fortunately, my experiences were not the same as Traweek's. Most of the time, I found myself in a position that was conducive to asking many questions. I have often found myself in what ethnographic textbooks refer to as an "apprentice role" where people have patiently answered my questions in detail. Sometimes my questions are strange and sometimes they even evoke a surprised expression or a smile, but these exact *moments of awkward encounters* might be moments where *friction* becomes visible, moments where different views and other aspects surface.[81]

Visitors to Turkey are immediately met with a warm hospitality. It seems like everybody you come across – even the police, who have a mixed reputation – see hospitality and helpfulness as the unquestioned mode of behaviour when someone visits their country, neighbourhood, farm, office, or when they step into the public vehicle they are driving. Everybody wants to help, and most of the time it is useful. Sometimes it can be a challenge though, to maintain a

76 Personal communication with two recovered avian influenza victims, Van 11. and12.06.2007

77 Personal communication with veterinary Ağrı Provincial Directorate of Agriculture and Rural Affairs, Ağrı 16.06.2007.

78 Personal communication with Prof. Dr. Ahment Faik Üner, Van University Hospital, 11.06.2007

79 Personal communication with Director of finances, poultry producing company, Balıkeşir 15.05.2007

80 Traweek, Sharon 1992

81 Tsing, Anna 2005

certain degree of independence and the personal space necessary to carry out research.

On one occasion, the two people who drove me to remote outbreak places in the eastern provinces became interested and highly engaged in the research. Apparently, they found it exciting to go to villages they would otherwise not have any reason to visit. As we arrived at the first village, they literary jumped out of the car before me. At the front of the building of the village administration, the two people enthusiastically introduced me to the staff, explaining my reason for visiting the village. We were immediately invited to the office of the head of administration. Joined by several other male staff members, we were served tea in accordance to Turkish customs. On the way to the office, my driver and his friend started chatting with the local civil servants and even asked some of them out. When we left the office, these "helpers" of mine asked me: "This was interesting for you, wasn't it?" In fact, I had not asked any questions; rather I had simply tried to follow the lively discussion between the six or seven men, as they walked in and out of the office. In order not to be impolite, I answered positively, but in fact, the biggest lesson learnt from this meeting was that I had to make our roles clear, and I had to find a way to do so without hurting anyone's feelings.

On this occasion, language was a problem. I was not able really to follow the intense discussions. I managed to ask permission to use a recorder, however, when I listened to the recording it was impossible to know who said what. Often several people talked at the same time, and for a long period, the most prominent sound was that of spoons being stirred in tea glasses surrounding the recorder that I strategically had put at the middle of the table. This is one of several sounds of Turkey; it triggers nostalgia and an eagerness to return. It is also the sound of a failed interview, which makes me smile as I look back, and which taught me a good lesson for the future.[82]

This situation was exceptional, however. Most of the time I talked with only one to three people at a time, and this early experience made me very much aware that I had to take the lead and make the roles clear if I arrived with someone else. My language skills are also both a good excuse and a reason for using a recorder. It sounds reasonable to say that I would like to use my recording machine so that I could listen to our talk again in case there was something I was unable to understand in the first place.[83]

---

82 This way of textualizing this event may well be seen in relation to Asdal's (2012) writing on context and the inter-relation between past, present and future that I will deal with in Chapter 5.

83 In "Writing Ethnographic Fieldnotes" the authors write about how making notes can some-

One surprising fact, which has made it easier to communicate with people in a foreign language, is that most of my informants have shown an impressive ability to realize when there were words I did not understand. They immediately took my signal – probably through a strange facial expression of my part – and repeated the word, found alternative words, or offered an explanation using short examples. During visits to villages, my rather simple language, together with all my other strangeness, might have contributed to removing the boundary between a "rich", "urban" and "well educated" stranger and themselves who are often regarded as ranging lower in the hierarchic Turkish society. My strange and basic questions were answered thoroughly and with patience.

Although it may sound naïve, it has been comfortable being a strange stranger in avian flu settings in Turkey; I have enjoyed hospitality, patience, helpfulness, confidence, and even forgiveness for strange behaviour stemming from being a stranger. Overall, I see it more as an advantage than a disadvantage. With respect to those who spend long periods *inside* the field "out there", continually possessing the role as the strange stranger, I can easily imagine that, in the long-term, it can become difficult and tiring.

## "There is no point of departure"

This chapter reflects on the main methodological resources and empirical material of this book – and not least how these are inseparable. It introduces the major "earthly relations",[84] "connections",[85] or "nodes"[86] which contribute in the becoming of the local and the national as well as the global avian influenza issue. Hence, the chapter discusses how empirical priorities and possibilities – or the modes of moving within the empirical field – are already influenced by the methodological modes I am moving around with. Positioning myself within STS, multi-sited fieldwork is acceptable, textual analyses are normal, and the combination is perhaps even potentially optimal – depending on the process and the effect, as this is being textualized, hence materialized, in the form of a book, and depending on the preferences of the reader. Simultaneously, the methods used are also being adjusted according to the empirical

times be an efficient way to make the informants feel important – when they see that you write they see that they tell you something of interest (Emerson, Robert, Rachel Fretz, and Linda Shaw 1995) My experience is that a record player can have the same effect.

84 Law, John and Annemarie Mol 2001, please also refer to the previous chapter.

85 Strathern, Marilyn 2004; Tsing, Anna 2005

86 Tsing, Anna 2005

field(s) along the way. In this way, this chapter presents and discuss the main analytical resources for this project.

The claim heading this final section, that "there is no point of departure", made a particular impression on me as I was struggling to work out how to start my fieldwork presentation; where did it begin? Massey quotes Louis Althusser, and the way I read him, with her, is that "there is nothing you have to accept as eternally pre-given, which is not in itself a product of previous causal structures."[87] Looking back at the point of "departure" of this chapter – which was actually the field notes on my *arrival* at a previous outbreak place – this might rather be seen as the opening of a path moving through and discussing various, but still connected, duals; I have discussed text-field, stability-flexibility, bio-geo and local-global.

Studying the intertwined and interactive relation between the methodology-empiric duality has enabled re-ordering various contributions from feminist techno-science, anthropology, sociology, history, and geology into a mode where these contributions are enacting complementary analytical resources in a way that allows them to realize each other's productive capacities. Alternatively, as Strathern has written with reference to the different parts of Haraway's cyborg: "they are realizing capacities for the other: each makes the other work".[88] As I have shown, Mol is carrying forth the same argument with regards to how *the body multiple* works.[89] In a similar vein, Moser, whose work I introduced in the previous chapter, is – through her practice-oriented studies of how people become and are made disabled, and also through her comprehensive studies on Alzheimer's disease – contributing to bringing out already existing, but often unrecognised or invisible alternatives to living with disabilities or Alzheimer's.[90] Moreover, Moser also emphasises how these relations may as well go in an opposite direction; that entities, versions, or what she often, like John Law, sees as modes of ordering, may not only contribute to make the other present; through her studies, she also highlights that one mode of ordering a matter of concern may contribute to making absence – to "disarticulate alternatives".[91] Finally, Asdal and Tsing show how interference or friction between two or more versions not only

87 Featherstone, David and Joe Painter 2013: 4 with reference to Massey, Doreen 1995: 351 who is referring to Althusser, Louis 1971: 85

88 Stathern, Marilyn 2004: 39

89 Mol, Annemarie 2002

90 See Moser, Ingunn 2005; Moser Ingunn 2008

91 See Moser, Ingunn 2008. Her argument with regards to making things absent and present and about disarticulating alternatives is of particular importance for my analysis in Chapter 6

results in realizing capacities for the other but also contributes to realizing something new.

Grasping the productive moment of these complimentary, rather than contradictory, contributions for studying the ordering, or becoming, and co-existence of heterogeneous realities offers the analytical tools to trace how heterogeneous objects may be realizing each other, how they may disarticulate each other, and how they together may contribute to realizing something new.

Re-writing this chapter over and over again, while simultaneously reading the work of others and re-viewing and re-thinking my analysis, has made me realize a vital duality that should not be neglected: that is the relation between reading and writing, re-reading and re-writing. Reflecting upon this makes me see how this text has moved in the process; some parts have changed more than others. It has become slightly longer, but mainly thicker; re-reading the works of others and re-thinking my own material, then re-formulating and re-writing has added layers to the text. As a result, perhaps the most central analytical concept or metaphor from previous drafts, *mobility,* is hardly mentioned in this version. That does not mean that it has lost its importance; indeed mobility is still present everywhere in this project; it is actively working within the layers of the text. All interactions, frictions, connections and relations that this book explores, is also about mobility. Moreover, the book aims to contribute to mobility; to influence the modes of ordering and to intervene in the formation of the avian influenza issue. One ambition is what Haraway terms "interference" and "diffraction", that is, to contribute in making difference.[92] My next interference will be to show how enacting matters of "biosecurity" relate to enacting bio*in*secutiry, and some of the effects thereof. That is the matter of concern for the next chapter.

[92] Law, John 1994. For a more explicit discussion on mobility in relation to this project, I refer to the previous introductory chapter.

# 3. Performing bioinsecurities

### Brandenburg, Germany 1709–1716[1]

In the early eighteenth century a serious epizootic outbreak affecting most of Europe threatened to destroy the cattle herds of the Hohenzollern Territory of Brandenburg in Northeast Germany. The danger to Brandenburg of an epidemic of a rinderpest-like cattle disease, between 1709 and 1716, stemmed mostly from the eastern European territories of East Prussia and of Poland. The disease, probably of Asian origin, was carried from southern Russia to Baltic and Central Europe by Swedish and Russian troops. In a decade of time the disease swept westward and reduced the cattle herds of Europe in the order of several million. To a large extent the threat to the cattle herds of Brandenburg from this epidemic was warded off by the first efforts at a scientific approach to the problem of cattle disease between 1711 and 1732.[2] The rinderpest-like epizooty (...) was spreading westward into Pomerania and Brandenburg. The threat of general epidemic to the cattle herds of Brandenburg resulted in the ordering of stringent protective measures by King Frederick I on 7 December 1711.[3]

### Balıkesir, Turkey 2005[4]

The continuing outbreaks of highly pathogenic avian influenza (HPAI), which begun in late 2003 in several Southeast Asian countries (...) have occurred more recently in parts of Europe(...).[5] To date Turkey has experienced one outbreak of avian influenza, in the Manyas district of Balikesir province. This outbreak was detected on October 1, 2005 when three turkeys died in a flock of 1,800 turkeys being raised by a medium sized poultry contract farmer in an outdoor grazing environment facility three kilometres south of Manyas Lake. This lake is a natural habitat for migratory birds, which were abundantly present at the time. Most of the rest of the flock died over the next three days, during which time the district veterinary service and a private veterinarian working for the poultry sector developed the diagnosis of avian influenza. Dead and live animals were sent to the Bornova reference laboratory (in Izmir), which detected the presence of the H5 strain (...). The EU reference laboratory in Weybridge (UK) confirmed the presence of the HPAI H5N1 strain on October 13.

---

1 Dorwart, Reinhold A. 1959

2 The text before this footnote is taken from *op. cit.*: 79, from here to the end of quote *op. cit*: 80

3 In the original text, Dorwart here includes a footnote referring to Mylius, Christian Otto (Ed.) 1740

4 Government of Turkey 2005 Dec.

5 This first part is taken from Ibid: Section 1c; the rest of the text is taken from Ibid: Section 1c

*Prevention and Isolation.* Among the first precautions ordered was a quarantine plan. No horn-beast was to be shipped into Brandenburg from Poland, Silesia or East Prussia unless it had been in quarantine for eight days on the borders. If none died in that period the cattle were to be allowed to pass. In East Prussia the seller of cattle was required to possess an affidavit that the place of origin of the cattle had been free of disease for three months. The epidemic continued to be serious for a number of years and the new king, Frederick William I, in 1714 and 1716[6], reaffirmed the shipping restrictions of 1711 in order "to prevent the ruin of the land." ( … ) Cattle markets in Brandenburg were closed. ( … ) If the disease could not be kept beyond the frontiers by quarantine or controlled import, the next step was to attempt to isolate it ( … ). By the Edict of 1711, the King's subjects were forbidden to place in common pasturage any cattle which were unhealthy or suspected of disease. ( … ) [T]he neighbours were permitted to keep such suspected cattle from the fields, or if the owner persisted in pasturing them, to shoot them and to bury them at once.

Sanitary measures had been promptly initiated by the provincial veterinary service on October 7, when a three kilometres protection zone was established with road sings and the presence of the military police. All backyard poultry (over 10,000 head) within the protection zone [were culled] between October 8–16, and compensation was granted by the private poultry industry itself to the affected farmers. Within the protection zone, there were also nine larger commercial holdings, seven of which were empty. The flock of almost 16,000 in the remaining two enterprises was slaughtered on October 9. In addition to the protection zone, a 10 km radius surveillance zone was established, which contained roughly 45,000 backyard poultry, and 10 active larger poultry farms with a stock of over 130,000 animals. Measures taken in the surveillance zone included a ban on the movement of live poultry, regulation of the transport of table and hatching eggs, prohibition of bazaar market trade of poultry and of hunting of wild birds, and an immediate local awareness campaign to instruct farmers to confine backyard poultry and avoid contact with wild birds.

The story of encounters with a rinderpest-like epizootic disease in the 18th century in Brandenburg, is told by historian Reinhold A. Dorwart in an article published in *Agricultural History* in 1959. The more recent story, about high pathogenic avian influenza (HPAI) H5N1 entering Europe and Turkey in 2005, is the official Turkish version conveying the status of the outbreak situation. This latter story is taken from the project appraisal submitted by the Turkish Ministry of Agriculture and Rural Affairs and the Ministry of Health to the World Bank (WB) in December 2005. The Turkish authorities sought financial

6 Again, Dorwart has a footnote referring to Mylius, Christian Otto (Ed.) 1740

support for the project, "Avian influenza and human pandemic preparedness and response". Dorwart's account on cattle disease hitting Germany should be seen as a historical account in a double sense: It was written nearly 70 years ago and it recollect events that took place more than 200 years earlier (now, more than 300 years ago). My intention is not to make this a historical chapter. However, I was struck by the Brandenburg story, given my research pertaining to ongoing measures to combat contemporary avian influenza outbreaks. The Brandenburg story serves as a reminder that the fight against animal diseases, and attempts to control nature, are not new; moreover, it highlights that our approach to addressing the issue is not so fundamentally different from the past.

In both of the above cases, Asia is pointed out as the place of origin for the disease. Furthermore, despite taking place in the $18^{th}$ century, the earlier story highlights that a "scientific approach to the problem" was crucial in terms of warding off the epidemic. Similarly, scientific methods, or tests carried out in specially approved national and international laboratories, confirmed veterinarians' suspicions that the disease they observed in the Manyas district of Turkey in 2005 was caused by HPAI virus of the H5N1 strain. While reading that King Frederick I was "ordering stringent control measures", we get the sense that this story is taking place in distant times; the *king's orders* offer the story an ancient and exotic touch. More specifically, the King "ordered (...) a quarantine plan", established "shipping restrictions", closed off cattle markets, and ordered the separation of healthy and unhealthy animals on pasturages. These specific measures or "attempts to isolate" the disease, as Dorward writes, relate closely to the "sanitary measures (...) initiated by" the more up-to-date sounding "provincial veterinary service" in Turkey during 2005. Measures mentioned in this latter text include establishing protection and surveillance zones, banning the movement of live poultry and transport regulations: "prohibition of bazaar market trade of poultry and instruct[ions to] farmers to confine backyard poultry".

The fact that the measures implemented in Balıkesir, Turkey in 2005 echoes those carried out in Brandenburg, Germany in 1711, as they were retold by Dorwart in the late 1950's, does not mean that the avian influenza outbreak in Turkey was handled in an old fashioned manner. On the contrary, the measures mentioned were in accordance with up-to-date international recommendations set out by the international institutions responsible for taking the lead in international efforts against transboundary animal diseases (TADs):

the World Organization for Animal Health (OIE) and the Food and Agriculture Organization of the United Nations (FAO).[7]

Both cattle plague and the measures against it have strong linkages to current international disease prevention work. According to Dorwart, it is uncertain whether it actually was rinderpest that hit Brandenburg at the beginning of the 18th century. However, in his investigations of the available material, which offered him an insight into the symptoms the farmers were faced with, he saw strong resemblances to this disease.[8] Rinderpest has recently been described as "the most dreaded bovine plague known, [and it] belongs to a select group of notorious infectious diseases that have changed the course of history."[9] It was an outbreak of this disease in Europe in 1920 that led to the establishment of the Office International des Epizooties, now also known as World Organization for Animal Health, (OIE).[10] Moreover, rinderpest was the disease at issue when the FAO Subcommittee on Animal Health issued its first recommendation in 1947.[11] In 2011, the OIE and the FAO declared that rinderpest had been eradicated, however these organizations still have other diseases to fight, and new diseases are frequently emerging.[12] Highly pathogenic avian influenza is one example of these new diseases.

This chapter is about biosecurity. But, but how do the two stories opening this chapter relate to biosecurity? The term is not explicitly mentioned in any of them. However, the practices mentioned in both of the stories fit one definition at work within the FAO, the OIE and the WHO: "The concept, [biosecurity,] preventing the spread of virus from infected premises (bio-containment), and measures requiring the exclusion of infectious agents from uninfected premises (bio-exclusion)".[13] The measures mentioned in the two stories above do just this; they aspire to prevent the mobility of the virus and to separate infected and uninfected spaces.

In relation to current disease control, the concept of *biosecurity* has become increasingly common. It is therefore worth paying special attention to this concept and this chapter is doing so. Firstly, the chapter will explore the increasing number of studies on this subject and it will examine some of the ways the concept is being used by the FAO and the OIE. Offering a compre-

7 See FAO 2004 Sept.
8 Dorwart, Reinhold A. 1959
9 Scott, Gordon R. and Alain Provost 1992: 1
10 Vallat, Bernard 2011
11 Scott, Gordon R. and Alain Provost 1992: 7
12 Vallat, Bernard 2011; OIE 2011
13 FAO, OIE and WHO 2005: 12; Nov. 2005: 16; Ivanov, Yanko 2007: 58

hensive overview on this issue is outside the scope of this project. Rather, I will introduce and discuss some contributions especially relevant for my own approach to biosecurity and to this book. Given the complexities of biosecurity, and the need for some kind of order when researching and writing about this subject, this chapter handle biosecurity as a matter of multiplicity, space and governance. Finally, I will examine the rather neglected relational nature of the concept by discussing how biosecurity is closely interrelated to what I will simply coin bio*in*security. In this respect, I will draw on the Turkish Ministry of Agriculture's report on the first reported outbreak of avian influenza in Turkey in order to trace how bio*in*security as well as biosecurity are ordered in the report. Drawing on the performative, processual and relational approaches introduced in the two first chapters of this book, I will study how this outbreak report contributes in order*ing* avian influenza.[14] I will also briefly explore how this ordering of an outbreak involves inclusion and exclusion, and the making of absence and presence in ways that contribute to enacting particular versions of bio(*in*)security.[15] For the purpose of the current chapter – which is primarily to address the importance of conceptualizing bio*in*security as a relational term to biosecurity – I will carry out a rather simple analysis, primarily based on textual analysis, but also juxtaposing text and the field "out there".[16] More extensive empirical analyses will be given in the following chapters where I will also introduce complementary analytical resources in a way that intends to add layers to both the empirical and analytical matters. As will be evident throughout this book, in addition to demonstrating the importance of bios*in*ecurity for biosecurity, I also seek to highlight that the way matters of bio(*in*)security have been ordered by responsible authorities in their reporting of this first outbreak of HPAI in Turkey, have impacted the ordering of future outbreaks.

## The introduction and spread of biosecurity

Andrew Donaldson and David Wood traced the first time the term biosecurity was mentioned in the British House of Commons as being on April 9, 2001.[17] In particular, British scholars within the field of science and technology studies (STS) have directed attention on how the spread of the term *biosecurity*

[14] Law, John 1994

[15] See especially Hinchliffe, Steve, John Allen, Stephanie Lavau, Nick Bingham and Simon Carter 2012, but on absence and presence more generally, please also refer e.g. to Asdal, Kristin 2007; Law, John and Annemarie Mol 2001; Moser, Ingunn 2008

[16] For a more thorough discussion of methodological approaches, please refer to Chapter 2.

[17] Donaldson Andrew and David Wood 2004: 373–374, with reference to Hansard 2001

within popular language, policy making and academic fields can be seen as a side effect of the severe food crisis that struck the Western world at the beginning of the new millennium. Media coverage of disastrous animal disease outbreaks, such as bovine spongiform encephalopathy (BSE), foot and mouth disease (FMD) and HPAI, in particular the H5N1 variant, contributed to distribution and spread of the term among the public.[18]

A report from the FAO's Committee on Agriculture meeting held in April 2003, stated that *"[b]iosecurity* is a relatively new concept and a term that is evolving as usage varies among countries with different specialist groups using it in different ways."[19] Steve Hinchliffe and Nick Bingham offer an overview of the various uses of the concept in their frequently cited article titled "Mapping the Multiplicities of Biosecurity". While they do not claim their "mapping" to be complete, it nevertheless provides a good impression of just the multiplicities of biosecurity.[20]

### Attending to the multiplicities of biosecurity

In short, Hinchliffe and Bingham's overview shows how biosecurity is being used in three different, yet interrelated settings that can roughly be traced to different parts of the world. Firstly, according to Hinchliffe and Bingham, the European emergence of biosecurity is seen "primarily in relation to attempts to manage the movement of agricultural pests and diseases."[21] Secondly, in Australia, New Zealand, remote islands and other places where in particular ecological colonization and introduction of species and farming systems, which were mainly initiated by European colonial powers, have come in conflict with local biodiversity concerns, biosecurity has come to refer to "efforts to reduce the effects of so-called invasive species on 'indigenous' flora and fauna."[22] Thirdly, Bingham and Hinchliffe's account brings us to the United States (US) where, as they point out, "biosecurity has come to represent a governmental concern with the – either purposeful or inadvertent – spreading of biological agents into the human populations".[23] They identify three areas where the US

[18] See e.g. Enticott, Gareth 2008; Donaldson, Andrew and David Wood 2004; Nerlich, Brigitte and Nick Wright 2006; Lakoff, Andrew and Stephen J. Collier (Eds.) 2008

[19] FAO 2003 April: Item 9 on the provisional agenda: point 2

[20] Bingham, Nick and Steve Hinchliffe 2008

[21] *Ibid.*: 173

[22] Bingham, Steve and Nick Hinchliffe 2008: 17. See also Barker, Kezia 2008; Lien, Marianne 2005

[23] *Op. cit.*

biosecurity approach is present: "[P]articular attention [is] given to laboratories that handle potentially hazardous organisms; possible use of pathogens in bioterrorism; and the prospect of animal-borne diseases [epizooties] crossing to humans (zoonoses)."[24] Social science or humanity based studies of biosecurity anchored in the US and/or focussing on US conditions often reflect the governmental system in which they are located. In US biosecurity studies, national security and defence aspects are intertwined with human and/or non-human health issues more so than in Europe.

Bingham and Hinchliffe warn against any efforts or attempts that seek to formulate and implement a one-size-fits-all-definition of biosecurity.[25] I tried to do this when I first began this project and strived to grasp the meaning of *biosecurity.* Apparently, biosecurity referred to specific practices, however further details were rarely specified. Sometimes, biosecurity has been explicitly mentioned or exemplified by hinting at (lack of) housing or fencing related to poultry hold. Other times the word, biosecurity, came up in relation to spraying disinfectants on cars entering the premises of poultry factories or exiting outbreak villages. Apparently, biosecurity was a major concern in relation to ornithologists sampling wild birds as part of active surveillance work, namely testing apparently healthy birds for possible viral infections. I understood that wild birds were perceived as a threat to biosecurity in that they could potentially introduce a virus to domestic poultry. Consequently, biosecurity was mentioned in relation to concerns regarding the sampling process when weather conditions and a lack of trained personnel were mentioned as common challenges towards biosecurity. In respect to the latter, I also heard about "cross-contamination" and possibly mixing of samples and insufficient tagging. I was unsure if these problems are considered matters of biosecurity.

Failing to understand exactly what biosecurity *is* and what it embraces, I have come to realize, particularly with the help of Bingham and Hinchliffe's research, but also via other literature, that it is necessary to attend to the multiplicities of biosecurity, and to attend to the practices through which biosecurity is being performed.

### Biosecuring – practices give content to the word and make disease outbreak visible

For more than a decade, scalars have been paying considerable attention to biosecurity and the practices through which biosecurity is performed. As men-

24 *Op. cit.*

25 Bingham, Nick and Steve Hinchliffe 2008

tioned above, Donaldson and Wood, among others, argue that the use of the term biosecurity increased during the 2001 European FMD epidemic.[26] They emphasise how "[British p]ig farmers may have understood its meaning after the procedures that they were encouraged to follow after the classical swine fever epidemic of the previous year (. . . )".[27] In other words, they show how practices carried out in the name of biosecurity have given content and meaning to the word; the practical expression of the concept of *biosecurity* came to reflect a relation to the disease and to the responses that were considered suitable to combat it. Further, they discuss biosecurity as a means of surveillance and intimidation.

While Donaldson and Wood focus on how specific procedures and practices have shaped the understanding of the concept biosecurity, Brigitte Nerlich and Nick Wright focus on the relation between practices and the disease. The authors' argue, "[f]or many," biosecurity measures such as "cleansing and disinfecting*became* Foot and Mouth".[28] In this way, "[b]iosecutity actions became invested with symbolic values and, in particular, where ritualised as part of the symbolic spatial construction of an otherwise 'invisible' enemy".[29] In other words, biosecurity measures contributed to making the disease real; invisible pathogens became visible through the biosecurity measures performed to eradicate it.

Nerlich and Wright's work is also drawing attention to how biosecurity measures are considered to be complied with in a good or bad manner and how this was used to deflect blame. Donaldson and Wood find that biosecurity has become a "banner of good practice for farmers" and that referring to biosecurity works as a "way of shifting the blame for the government's failing in disease management onto farmers".[30] Farmers interviewed in Nerlich and Wright's study "talked about biosecurity measures in ways other than just reducing risk; they became a focus for the construction of coping strategies and attempts to lay blame and to resist blame".[31] In the same vein, Gareth Enticott points out that "[farmers were] accused of poor farming in that they had not implemented the recommended biosecurity measures. However," he emphasises, in line with Nerlich and Wright among others, that "the report into the

26 Donaldson, Andrew and David Wood 2004

27 Donaldson, Andrew and David Wood 2004:382

28 Nerlich, Brigitte and Nick Wright 2006: 441, *italics in original.*

29 *Op. cit*

30 Donaldson Andrew and David Wood 2004: 373

31 Nerlich, Brigitte and Nick Wright 2006: 458

2001 FMD outbreak also suggested that many of the recommended biosecurity measures(…) were futile exercises."[32]

By attending to practices through which biosecurity is performed, these studies also show how biosecurity is perform*ing*; particular efforts to control a specific disease have given content and meaning to the concept biosecurity. Biosecurity measures have made the disease visible and real; moreover, biosecurity measures work as a means of surveillance, intimidation and for placing blame on various actors. Reflecting on how biosecurity is often used in highly performative ways, Nick Bingham and Steve Hinchliffe suggest using the verb "*biosecuring* – a verb that [they] prefer to the noun 'biosecurity' in that it highlights the unfinished business of making safe".[33] In this regard, our attention should be directed towards at least three interrelated areas of *unfinished business*: the making of how to make safe – that is the identification of the nature of the problem and the suitable solutions thereof, and the business of putting these solutions or measures into practice.

## Biosecurity and spatiality

Donaldson and Wood engage a broad definition of biosecurity as a "technical concept ( … ) that refers principally to a set of simple procedures intended to prevent coincidental spread of disease through normal activities".[34] Similar to Donaldson and Woods, Enticott takes a spatial or geographical approach to biosecurity when he examines "new attempts to encourage farmers to purify agricultural space by 'building out' disease"[35]. While Donaldson and Wood referred to "simple procedures" like hand washing, Enticott focuses on "physical barriers" aiming "to divide space into healthy and infectious zones" as a means of preventing the transmission of infectious agents.[36] While Enticott focuses on "the mobility of disease *within* agricultural space (that is, individual farms)"[37] others have examined government attempts to – or failure to – prevent spread "*between* agricultural spaces (at local, national and international scales)".[38] In

---

32 Enticott, Gareth 2008: 1568. Here he also refers to Nerlich, Brigitte and Nick Wright 2006 and NFU in BBC 2007 (BBC, 2007 *Farming Today* This Week, Radio 4, 11 August)

33 Hinchliffe, Steve and Nick Bingham 2008b: 1542

34 Donaldson, Andrew and David Wood 2004: 373

35 Enticott, Gareth 2008: 1569

36 Donaldson, Andrew and David Wood 2004: 373; Enticott, Gareth 2008: 1569

37 Enticott, Gareth 2008: 1569, *emphasis in original.*

38 Continue paraphrasing Enticott, *op.cit*. Some other crucial contributions are Hinchliffe, Steve 2001; Law, John and Annemarie Mol 2006; Nerlich, Brigitte and Nick Wright 2006; Donaldson, Andrew and David Wood 2004.

the *Global Strategy for the Progressive Control of Highly Pathogenic Avian Influenza (HPAI)*, which I will discuss in the next two chapters, "the application of biosecurity measures" is emphasised as "[o]ne of the most important aspects of HPAI control and prevention". Here biosecurity is about flows in two directions; it is about "prevention of spread of virus from infected premises (bio-containment) and measures requiring the exclusion of infectious agents from uninfected premises (bio-exclusion)."[39]

As my analysis in the next two chapters will show, a major matter of concern highlighted in the Global Strategy and in the related Turkish National Strategy, is how already existing high pathogenic viruses are moving to new places. It is about *spread* and I will trace what Hinchliffe et al. call a *topographic approach* or a "linear and one-way transfer story of avian influenzas".[40] Writing against such linear transfer stories, Hinchliffe et al. advocate for a move to topology, to particular networked approaches that provide space for complexity in ways that are offering the robustness necessary for handling indeterminate events, such as disease outbreaks. Crucially, Hinchliffe et al. do not perceive networks as fixed, but as unstable and indeterminate, and as being made up of complex and changing relations and interferences. Such an approach may offer a more suitable way of dealing with the *multiplicities of biosecurity* and the indeterminate and relational matters of avian influenza.

The studies briefly examined here and the Global Strategy all illustrate how biosecurity works to conceptualize the flow of infective agents in various directions: in, out, within and between and through linear as well as networked spaces. A topological network approach is offering space for far more complex relations and "intra-actions", some of which will be further explored in this and later chapters.[41] What I will draw from this for now, is that biosecurity is about movement, flows and circulations. As Hinchliffe and Bingham argue, biosecurity is about good and bad circulations.[42]

## Biosecurity: a holistic concept governing human, animal and plant life globally

Biosecurity is a strategic and integrated approach that encompasses the policy and regulatory frameworks (including instruments and activities) that analyse and manage

39 FAO, OIE and WHO 2005 May: 12; Nov: 16; Ivanov, Yanko 2007: 58

40 Hinchliffe, Steve and Nick Bingham 2008b: 1543

41 Hinchliffe, Steve, John Allen, Stephanie Lavau, Nick Bingham and Simon Carter 2012: 7. They are here drawing on Karen Barad's (2007) term "intra-act".

42 Hinchliffe, Steve and Nick Bingham 2008b

risks in the sectors of food safety, animal life and health, and plant life and health, including associated environmental risk. (... )*Biosecurity* is a holistic concept of direct relevance to the sustainability of agriculture, food safety, and the protection of the environment, including biodiversity.[43]

This definition of "*Biosecurity*" appears on the FAO's website, on a page titled "Priority Areas for Inter-disciplinary Action (PAIAs)". In this text, biosecurity is more than just the sum of simple practices for separation, inclusion and exclusion; it is "a strategic and integrated approach"; it is "instruments", "activities", "analysis" and "management". Further research reveals that biosecurity is also "information exchange"[44] and an "international policy and regulatory framework"[45]. This shows how biosecurity becomes a tool kit for governance of agriculture, food and the environment *globally*.

The FAO's definition of "*Biosecurity*" embraces all the three fields highlighted in Bingham and Hinchliffe's mapping of the multiplicities of biosecurity: agricultural disease and pest control, protection against invasive species, and intended or unintended spread of potential hazardous organisms. The FAO's Committee on Food and Agriculture has also identified a long list of "[b]inding international legal instruments relevant to biosecurity in food and agriculture" which also includes forestry and fishery.[46] Some examples are the International Plant Protection Convention (IPPC), the Constitution of the European Commission for the Control of Foot and Mouth Disease, The World Trade Organization's (WTO) Agreement on the Application of Sanitary and Phytosanitary Measures (SPS Agreement), the Biological Weapons and Toxins Convention, the Convention on Biological Diversity and its Cartagena Protocol on Biosafety, the United Nations Convention on the Law of the Sea, and the Ramsar Convention on Wetlands. Furthermore, this integrated approached

[43] http://www.fao.org/biosecurity/, italics in original, *read 16.08.2014.* FAO's Committee in Agriculture recommended that, due to "translation challenges", especially for Spanish and French, the English term *Biosecurity* is not translated but italicized and capitalized: "Following considerable discussion on terminology, delegates agreed that the term *Biosecurity* in food and agriculture best describes the concept as used by FAO(... )" (FAO 2003 April: point 25). In Turkish, the word *biyogüvenlik* is used for both biosecurity and biosafety (for example in the Turkish version on the Cartangena Protocol on Biosafety, *Cartagena Biyogüvenlik Protokolü*). While the English version of the Turkish National Strategy (Ivanov, Yanko 2007) uses both biosecurity and biosafety, where the latter applies to matters related to laboratories and vaccines, the Turkish version of this document exclusively uses *biyogüvenlik,* which covers both *biosecurity* and *biosafety.*

[44] FAO 2003 April: Item 9 on the provisional agenda: point 15

[45] FAO 2001 March: Item 8 on the provisional agenda: point 16

[46] *Op. cit*: point 13

is materialized by various documents produced in collaboration between the FAO, the OIE and the WHO, such as global strategies for avian influenza control; this will be thoroughly studied in the following two chapters. These examples offer an impression of the wide reaching "integrated approach" and "multi-sectorial" diversity tied together by the "holistic concept" of "*Biosecurity*".

While central practices of biosecurity resemble century old practices of hygiene and sanitation, it can be suggested that the practices are made novel by the "multi-sectorial" institutionalization and "integrated approach",aiming to govern "globally" across fields and territories that have previously been governed more separately.[47] In 2007, the FAO published a so-called Biosecurity Tool Kit in order to provide "practical guidance and support to develop and implement national biosecurity frameworks at the country level."[48] The explicitly addressed "target audience" primarily included "government officials ( . . . ) involved in food safety and public health, animal and plant life and health, and protection of the environment, at both the policy and/or operational level", but also "development agencies, consultants and trainers supporting biosecurity activities and programmes."[49] This is just one example of how the FAO attempted to influence institutionalization on a national level in the name of biosecurity.

Natalie Porter's study on health cadres in Vietnam contests this top-down approach. Rather than simply turning to counter approaches advocating grass root initiatives or bottom-up approaches, Porter contributes to sustaining what she refers to as "recent theories of governmentality that reject binary distinctions between transnational development frameworks and state governing techniques".[50] Through her ethnographic study, Porter shows how international recommendations for behavioural change which aim to increase the levels of biosecurity as a means of disease prevention and control, were played out in a melange of an international script for a simulation exercise and various national communist elements in a local setting. Hence, recommendations from the top are not simply transferred to and implemented on the ground. Porter argues that "[o]n the ground" they were made Vietnamese and the local health cadre in charge "enacted global health agendas by utilizing established national mobilization practices". Moreover, by displaying successful work, this event –

47 FAO n. d., *italics in original*

48 FAO 2007

49 FAO 2007: xi

50 Porter, Natalie 2013: 92, with reference to Agrawal, Arun 2005; Li, Tania Murray 2007; Ong, Aihwa 2006

the simulation exercise – was working simultaneously as a tool for securing further project funding for "on the ground" projects from the foreign for-profit organization whose representatives attended the exercise, and as a practice of biosecure behaviour as described or advised international organizations "at the top".

According to my analysis in this section, biosecurity is about institutionalization and governance. Porter's study shows that biosecurity, as an element of heterogeneous "global health" interventions, is more than demands from "above" and/or "resistance" from "below"; biosecurity is complex and a matter of negotiation. What this study is not addressing though, is how matters and practices come to be regarded as biosecure in the first place. That is a matter of concern for this volume. In order to study this, it is now time to address the relational nature of the term biosecurity.

## The importance of risk for security

Although still rather neglected in social science studies, the term *biosecurity* assumes that these various forms of life, *bio*, need to be *secured*; it implicitly claims that there must be something to secure *from* or *against*, or as these various FAO texts make clear, that bio*security* is connected to *risk:*

**FAO, Committee on Biosecurity in Food and Agriculture:**

> *Biosecurity* involves the management of biological *risks* in a comprehensive manner ( . . . ) *Risk analysis*[51] is the most important unifying concept across different *Biosecurity* sectors.[52]

**FAO Biosecurity Tool Kit:**

> Biosecurity is a strategic and integrated approach to analysing and managing relevant *risks* to human, animal and plant life[1] and health and associated *risks* to the environment.[53]

**FAO and OIE: Biosecurity for Highly Pathogenic Avian Influenza:**

> Biosecurity is the implementation of measures that reduce the *risk* of the introduction and spread of disease agents. Biosecurity requires the adoption of a set of attitudes and behaviours by people to reduce *risk* in

51 "Risk analysis as used in this document includes risk assessment, risk management and risk communication, unless otherwise indicated", footnote to FAO 2003 April: point 26.

52 FAO 2003 April: point 26, *words boldfaced by me.*

53 FAO 2007: viii, X, 95*words boldfaced by me.*

> all activities involving domestic, captive exotic and wild birds and their products.[54]

The FAO Biosecurity Tool Kit, from where I have taken one of the texts above, primarily defines various hazards and provides "*[a]n overview and framework manual for biosecurity risk analysis*".[55] Based on my extensive studies of texts dealing with avian influenza I have noted that, more often than not, *biosecurity* is accompanied by possible biosecurity *risks* or potential biosecurity *hazards*. While bio*security* is enacted as the aim to reach, it soon becomes apparent that the focus is most often directed towards identifying, preventing and reporting risks and hazards – matters of *in*security. In her study on scientists of molecular biology, Susan Wright has shown how scientists escaped criticism by moving the attention away from the *risk* of releasing pathogens outside the lab towards laboratory *safety*.[56]

According to Wright's study, laboratory safety, often referred to as biosafety, worked as a means to make distance to or move the attention away from concerns in regards to risk. In relation to avian influenza, when biosecurity is the issue, the matter of concern is often the risks, threats and hazards towards life – this is what I call bio*in*securities.

When introducing the concept bio*in*security, it might be worthwhile to make a distinction between this and what Hinchliffe and Bingham and others are addressing as "insecurities of biosecurity" or "bio-insecurities".[57] They have used this term to address the possible negative external effects of interventions aiming to improve biosecurity; they highlight the "complex security issues" associated with intensive farming systems and point at "the ability of such systems to reproduce insecurities at the very same time they offer their solution."[58] By suggesting bio*in*security as a companion to biosecurity, my aim is to stress the importance of the relational capacities of bio(in)security. I argue that bio*in*security should receive explicit attention in a symmetrical way to biosecurity: In order to avoid taking the object of study for granted, studies of biosecurity need also to take bio*in*securities into account, and pay attention to the interplay between securities and insecurities.

---

54 FAO and OIE: Biosecurity for Highly Pathogenic Avian Influenza 2008:1, *words boldfaced by me.*

55 FAO 2007: title of section 3 of 3 (pp. 41–89)

56 Wright, Susan 1986

57 Hinchliffe, Steve and Nick Bingham 2008b

58 Hinchliffe, Steve and Nick Bingham 2008b: 1548

## How avian influenza outbreak contributes to enacting bio(in)security

Outbreak places are working well for studying how matters come to be enacted as threatening to life, as bio*in*secure. As pointed out in the previous chapter, a place becomes an outbreak place only after positive laboratory tests prove the presence of particular pathogen already decided upon as threatening and unwanted. Following from this, the current chapter argues that becoming an outbreak place is also becoming a site for bioinsecurity. I will return to the avian influenza outbreak that, together with the similar rinderpest outbreak, opened this chapter. As an outbreak place and a site for bio*in*security, it provides a strategic place for analysing how the threat to life – bio*in*security – is being enacted.

### "Information on the outbreak" I: Enacting a site as wild bird habitat

The initial outbreak of HPAI H5N1 in Turkey is discussed in a 24-page report submitted to the European Commission by the Republic of Turkey's Ministry of Agriculture and Rural Affairs General Directorate of Protection and Control. Before the outbreak is mentioned, the report provides an eight-page introduction and overview of the country. A general introduction immediately positions Turkey in relation to its neighbouring countries by listing these and the length of the shared borders, including the three coastal borders.

In addition to positioning Turkey in relation to its neighbouring countries, the general introduction also positions the country within four migratory routes, stating that, "four main routes of wild migratory bird are passing through over Anatolia."[59] The importance of wild birds for the general characteristic of the country is further strengthened by the following statement: "Turkey is one of the richest countries for having site areas [or important wild bird areas] in Europe and Middle East." This, coupled with the fact that "four main routes of wild migratory birds are passing through over Anatolia", contribute to enact wild birds as important actors all over the country. The general introduction continues by introducing one specific locality, Manyas Lake, a "renown wild bird reserve", which "harbours more than 250 different bird species", and "[i]t is estimated that up to 3 million birds in a year come to the lake."[60]

59 MARA 2005: 2

60 MARA 2005: 2

The second part of the introduction establishes Turkey as a poultry producing country. I will soon analyse this part too. However, first I will study the text where the outbreak first appears in this document: the ninth page of the 24-page report, under the heading *Disease Situation*.

On page nine, the wild bird reserve Manyas Lake, introduced at the very beginning of the report, reappears. Previously enacted as a particularly important site for wild birds, Lake Manyas here becomes the only relevant point of reference for the outbreak place. As Manyas Lake reappears in this section of the report; it becomes the scene of an outbreak of HPAI; the "renown wild bird reserve" is turned into a place of bio*in*security. The text makes it clear that the wild birds of Manyas Lake are a "likely" source. Indeed, they are the only likely source: "In the absence of any relevant tracing back contacts the hypothesis that the turkeys contracted the virus from wild birds ranging around the nearby Manyas Lake is a likely one."[61] The likeliness of this hypothesis is strengthened by information from a farm employee who has reportedly noted "frequent visits of wild quails (this is apparently a migratory species) to the rice fields where the turkeys were kept."[62] The fact that, "to date, no abnormal mortality or clinical problems have been observed in the wild bird populations staying on the lake" despite "good follow up system for the birds' populations on the lake", does not seem to alter the conclusion that wild and "apparently ( ... ) migratory" birds were the source of the infection. In this way, the "rich" wildlife habitat are turned into a "likely" – that is the *only* "likely" – source of infection; Manyas Lake and the present wild birds becomes a space for and a source of bio*in*security for domestic poultry in the area.

## "Information on the outbreak" II: Enacting a site as isolated agricultural land

The introduction of the outbreak report proceeds, after the presentation of the role of Turkey as an important wild bird area, with a short description of the national poultry industry. The poultry industry is enacted as a "well developed sector of agriculture in Turkey." Backyard poultry is only mentioned in general terms as being highly present "in the countryside". Even though "there is no exact number" on the backyard poultry population, it is referred to as "quite big". The indecipherable nature of backyard poultry is in contrast to commercial poultry where "[a]ll commercial flocks are registered." Other characteristics used to describe commercial poultry production are "modern and closed".

[61] MARA 2005: 11
[62] MARA 2005: 11

Furthermore, commercial flocks are stated to be "under ( . . . ) regular inspection and control", and, in addition to controls of integrated flocks by private veterinarians, "commercial flocks are [also] controlled by official veterinarians for usage of veterinary medicinal drugs, vaccinations, biosecurity measurements [?] and hygienic conditions and etc."[63] While backyard poultry is enacted as being outside of control, even in terms of numbers or extent, commercial poultry appears to be well controlled and integrated into some kind of biosecurity regime. To my knowledge, "biosecurity measurements" is an uncommon concept, resembling the frequently used *biosecurity measures*. No further specification is given regarding what these "measurements" involve. The reference to the term may be seen as an attempt to associate the sector with this positive loaded term, biosecurity, which commonly represent a goal to reach, a solution and a prerequisite to successful disease control.

Furthermore, the introduction relates backyard poultry hold to "the country side", the general introductory presentation contributes to position the majority of the 16.701 commercial flocks "in western part of Turkey." It should be noted that Manyas district and Manyas Lake are located in the western part of Turkey; however, this is not mentioned and no explicit relation is made between the outbreak place and the area of Turkey where the majority of commercial poultry production is located. Instead, it is explicitly mentioned that the few *semi-closed* farms that exist are in the Mediterranean and Aegean region. As *closed* is a precondition for good biosecurity, and *open* is associated with low or no biosecurity, semi-closed does also, in this setting, imply questionable biosecurity conditions. The report specifies that these farms, with questionable biosecurity conditions, are located relatively far away from the outbreak places; thus, according to the report, they are situated in other areas and not present in the outbreak area. No further details are given regarding the poultry sector in the outbreak area. While wild bird habitats are made a relevant characteristic of Lake Manyas, no such connection is made between the lake or the surrounding land and domestic poultry production in this report.

Furthermore, while the presentation of Turkey as a wild bird paradise is accompanied by two maps, one illustrating important wild bird habitats protected under the Ramsar Convention and the other illustrating the "Main Migration routes of wild birds", no maps, tables, or text provide any impression of main locations for poultry production. Nor does the report provide any impression of the network of poultry product trade routes, within or beyond the country. One table in the annexes (Annex 1) offers an overview of the"[n]umber of poultry

63 MARA 2005: 3, *italics added.*

species and chicken meat production". However, these numbers are country totals. While this table illustrates the growing importance of poultry production in the country *in general,* it does not make any connection between the commercial sector and the outbreak region in particular. This generalization of the poultry sector contributes to delocalizing the sector; any possible relation between outbreak place and the fast growing, intensive poultry production is thus avoided, ensuring that this form of domesticated life remains secure, in the sense of not associated with the outbreak.

In order to get an impression of how the infected turkey farm relate to other farming activities or other poultry hold in the area, we have to return to the description of the *Disease Situation* of the report. Here the report makes rhetorical efforts to literally isolate this outbreak from other commercial poultry activity in the area:

> The farm is *very isolated* from other poultry farms (both professional and backyard) in the area: on the north side the farmland (mainly rice fields) and grassland changes into the swampy shore of the [Manyas] lake, on the east side the farm is bordering farmland and a military practice ground, on the west side and south side the farm is surrounded by only farm land. The nearest professional poultry farm is situated in the village of Kiziksa to the southeast at about 2,5 km.[64]

This *Information on the outbreak* immediately separates the outbreak farm from other poultry farms. In a shorter outbreak report, the so-called *Immediate notification form*, sent from the national authorities to the OIE in accordance with procedures regarding the notification of animal diseases, the outbreak place appears even more isolated: "The outbreak occurred in a backyard flock kept in a sparsely populated area (military zone) between Kiziksa and Salur villages in Manyas district, Balikesir province."[65] However, a rather different picture emerges upon further examination of the document.

At the end of the text, a "professional poultry farm" emerges, well within the so-called 3 km radius protection zone from the outbreak place. In addition, another epidemiologically relevant space appears one and a half pages later: "The epidemiological inquiry revealed only one direct contact holding. Just prior to the onset of the clinical problems (...) another 2.684 turkeys ranging on the same grounds were separated and moved to a ground about 1 km away."[66] By ensuring that "all precautionary measures" were taken, that

---

64 MARA 2005: 9, *italics added.*

65 OIE Immediate Notification Report, reference: Ref OIE: 5306, Report Date: 10/10/2005, Country: Turkey, http://web.oie.int/wahis/reports/en_imm_0000005306_20051010_172322.pdf, *read 16.07.2014.*

66 MARA 2005: 11

"no relevant contacts" were made, and finally by ensuring the "absence of any clinical problem in the flock that was separated from the affected flock," the connection to this field is made irrelevant. As part of the "preventive culling", a central biosecurity measure and means of hindering virus circulation, these latter turkeys were reportedly culled. However, in relation to preventive culling, another "7.363 backyard poultry" does also appear within "the protection zone (3km)". Furthermore, the report reveals "2 broiler farms on the outskirts [one apparently mentioned above] of the protection zone and 2 broiler farms within the surveillance zone [further 3–10 km out from the outbreak centre] that all housed poultry".[67] While all the backyard poultry were culled, "[n]o professional poultry were culled."[68] The latter were slaughtered, and "[t] he meat was commercialised as fresh meat on the national market."[69] In the section describing the measures that had been taken, it becomes apparent that there is even more professional poultry hold within the protection zone. Seven professional poultry holdings appear here which had not previously been mentioned. These seven holdings were reportedly "empty", but the report provides no information why or for how long seven of nine poultry holdings were empty. The fact that they were empty does also indicate that it would not have been possible to test the poultry for possible infection that might possibly have been kept in these holding in the relevant and recent past. Further, in addition to the two holdings already mentioned in the surveillance zone the total number of holdings here appears to be 15. Together these housed 131.500 chickens and hens. Of these, five were "empty". Finally, 45.000 backyard poultry also appear in the surveillance zone.

The farm that initially was described as "very isolated" does not appear to be so isolated after all. However, no alternative hypothesis is set out to compete with the one stating that, "[i]n the absence of any relevant tracing back contacts the hypothesis that the turkeys contracted the virus from wild birds ranging around the nearby Manyas Lake is a likely one".[70]

67 The surveillance zone is the area in a 3–10 km radius around the outbreak centre. As mentioned above, the area within 3 km radius of the outbreak place is called protection zone. Various biosecurity measures apply to these two zones aiming at reducing the risk of spread (bio-inclusion). See FAO, OIE and WHO 2005 Mai; 2005 Nov.

68 MARA 2005: 11

69 MARA 2005: 11

70 MARA 2005: 11

## "Information on the outbreak" III: Wild-domestic interferences

Manyas district is indeed a well-known wild bird habitat, with Manya Lake and the adjacent national park, Kuş Cennetti, attracting ornithologists and bird enthusiasts from all over Turkey as well as from abroad. Furthermore, no matter from which direction one arrives in Balıkesir province, the presence of commercial poultry production is also very apparent; poultry houses are scattered all over the province, and along the highway towards Bursa and Izmir, travellers are passing feeding mills, slaughterhouses, and other buildings and trucks, which are obviously involved in poultry production as evidenced by their highly visible trademarks and billboards. Additionally, the local city centre of Bandırma is coloured by the presence of the two largest poultry producers in the area: by the harbour, kids enjoyed their time at the playground sponsored by one of them, Şeker Piliç, (as pictured below), and the modern Banvit Basketball Stadium, named after their main sponsor and leading poultry producer, provides ground for more serious games.

My plan was to interview employees working at one of the large poultry producing companies in the area, as well as to visit the outbreak village. My concerns about how to get to the reportedly remote outbreak village quickly dissipated when one of my informants from the poultry company offered to take me to some of their integrated farms. One of the farms he brought me to appeared to be located *in* the outbreak village, well within what had been defined as the 3 kilometre protection zone during the time of the outbreak.

The two geographical features of the Manyas area, namely, a wild bird habitat and an agricultural area, are both related to the area's good infrastructure. For the poultry industry, this means proximity to the highway, railway and strategic harbours. For the birds, it means special wind conditions making the nearby strait of Bosporus one of the world's best "bottlenecks" for bird migration, as soaring birds can ride the thermal streams on their seasonal journey. It is evident that wildlife and agriculture coexist in the Manyas area. However, this is not apparent in the outbreak report that documents HAPI in the area. No traffic routes are mentioned except for migratory flyways.

In order to gain a more detailed image of commercial poultry production, one has to move beyond the outbreak report, to venture into the field, or to study alternative texts. A report on Turkey, titled *Market Impacts of HPAI Outbreaks* ( … ) is for example turning Manyas into a district of intensive poultry production.[71] This report enacts the province of Bandirma, where Manyas district is located, as the country's second largest producer of egg and poultry.

[71] Yalcin, Cengiz 2006

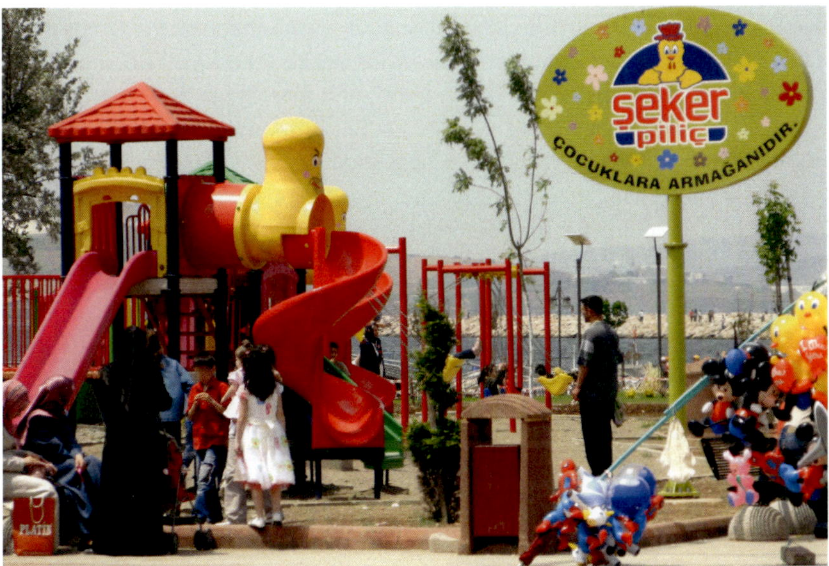


*Picture from fieldtrip to Bandırma, 15.05.2007. The playground, which is located centrally at the harbour area by the shore of lake Marmara, is sponsored by the poultry producer, Şeker Piliç.*

This market impact report shows how the poultry disease had severe consequences on the egg and white meat industry. The report does not explicitly address the pathological effects on the affected birds. Rather, it address the economical effects on the industrial poultry sector; in this report, avian influenza is causing a "market shock" as soon as the public became aware of the outbreak.[72]

In my interview with the director of finances at one of the above mentioned poultry companies the "market shock" version of avian influenza turned out to be complex. The director explained to me how his firm, like the other leading firms in the country, managed relatively well through the avian influenza crisis due to their capacity to freeze and store their products until the market recovered from the shock.[73] Moreover, the authorities' attempts, in relation to the initial avian influenza outbreak, to strengthen the control of poultry products by forbidding the bulk sale of poultry products and making packing and tagging obligatory, had a positive effect on this and other leading firms, un-

72 See e.g. Yalcin, Cengiz 2006

73 Personal communication with Director of finances, poultry producing company, Balıkeşir 15.05.2007

like the smaller ones. Prior to the outbreak of avian influenza, the larger firms had already established brands. Thus, when packing became obligatory, and branding consequently became more important, these large firms experienced yet another competitive advantage. The smaller firms often lacked the financial resources and equipment required to store products for better times, as well as for packing and changing their production line in accordance to new demands. Several firms could not afford to restart production after the crisis. The story told by the director of finances of this poultry firm goes well together with the findings of the market impact report, which concludes the following:

> [s]urvivors [of the initial outbreak of HPAI H5N1 and the countrywide spread the following winter], particularly those invested in brand development are likely to be better off in the future. Previously, consumption of commercial poultry meat and eggs by the rural families were negligible. However, as a result of ban on spent hen sales in local market, and depopulation of backyard poultry, the industry has been increasing their sales volumes in the rural markets.[74]

While some firms went bankrupt, others managed to turn the avian influenza crisis into an opportunity by taking advantage of the situation; the immediate costs related to the so-called market shock was paid back with increasing market share when the situation returned to normal.[75]

Attending to some of the specificities of Manyas district shows how this area offers more than just wetlands and wild bird habitats; it is also an area of intensive poultry production. Moreover, paying attention to how this market shock affected the commercial poultry sector shows how this sector is heterogeneous and how the various firms made it through the crisis with different results. This again must be seen in relation to how the outbreak was ordered as a wild bird issue; hence, free-range poultry were enacted as insecure lives, which in this case were the infected and affected turkey flock and backyard poultry.

Based on my analysis in this chapter, I will argue that by not being part of the outbreak area enacted in the outbreak report, the large scale commercial poultry sector remained secure; this sector, the sites of intensive poultry production and their market connections, remained *biosecure*; it was secured from being associated with pathogens, and the economic life of the sector was secured; the outbreak report contributed to separating the sector from the outbreak place in a way that kept it "clean", thus it suffers no long term negative economic effects. The negative economical effects were only short term, and

[74] Yalcin, Cengiz 2006: 4, 28

[75] See also Yalcin, Cengiz 2006

thus devastating for the smaller producers, not the larger ones.[76] In this way, exclusion did not have a marginalizing effect on the largest producers; rather it has an empowering effect.

Furthermore, as the outbreak report explicitly states, no wild birds were identified as being infected. However, through the bird's migratory flyways and their habitat in wetlands, they were given the role as *the only* "possible source" of infection. In this way, the report enacts a relation between domestic turkeys and wild birds; while wild birds were not found to be infected, they were affected in the way that they and their migratory flyways and habitats became matters of bio*in*security.

## Drawing the multiplicities of bio(in)securities together

This chapter has explored the concept of biosecurity, partly in relation to the initially reported outbreak of HPAI caused by the H5N1 virus strain in Turkey that was detected in the Manyas district, located in the north-western province of Balıkesir, in October 2005. In order to do so, I have organized biosecurity as a matter of multiplicity, space and governance. My main contribution to studies of biosecurity has been to attend to how biosecurity is closely interrelated to bio*in*security. By coining this concept, I intend to emphasise how bio*in*security deserves explicit attention, as this is more often than not what biosecurity is actually about. Bio*security* is interrelated to the threats, risks and hazards to safe living; thus, when a disease outbreak occurs, it is bio*in*security that is at stake.

In her study on laboratories and the risk of releasing hazardous waste, Wright showed how scientists have avoided critiques by focussing less on *risk* and more on laboratory *safety*. Similarly, I have traced how the report from the Ministry of Agriculture on the initial HPAI (H5N1) outbreak in Turkey have made risk, or more precisely bio*in*security, the main matter of concern; consequently, by keeping other matters out, these remain matters of biosecurity.

My analysis of the Ministry of Agriculture's report on the first reported avian influenza outbreak in Turkey shows how wild birds have been made a likely source of infection of domestic turkeys. Furthermore, when they are not just a likely source, but *the only* likely source, avian influenza spread come to be enacted as moving exclusively from wild to domestic. By focusing on identifying the source of infection, the report contributes to making bio*in*security a

76 For a further analysis on the socioeconomic impacts, especially in regard to contracting farmers in Turkey, see Yalcin, Cengiz 2006 and Geerlings, Ellen 2006.

matter of concern. Wild birds, and possible connections between wild and domestic birds, have become matters of bio*in*security. Commercial poultry production has been kept out or literally removed from the report in ways that avoid associating this sector with the outbreak. This separation was necessary to make wild birds the only likely source, but at the same time, it also ensured that the commercial sector remained biosecure. Similarly, Hinchliffe and Bingham stress how the imagined unilinear spread of avian influenza "from wild birds to domestic birds and from farm animals to humans invites its own version of disease risk ( . . . ) it generates its own strategies for interventions".[77] This is a vital argument for my book too. Hence, I am expanding upon Hinchliffe and Bingham's advice to stay attentive to how topology and direction are being enacted in ways that may call for interventions which could potentially lead to situations that make life insecure rather than more secure; my analysis stresses how interventions advocated in the name of biosecurity may lead to what Hinchliffe and Bingham, in their later work together with others, refer to as "intra-actions that make disease a possibility in the first place".[78]

This study of how this initial outbreak among turkeys in Turkey has been ordered in the official outbreak investigation report shows how the report enacts a particular topology of bio*in*security. Moreover, a detailed analysis and juxtaposing of this report with other sites at where Manyas district is being enacted shows how this particular topology involves separation, and that other matters too could have become matters of bio*in*security. This particular way of ordering bio*in*security, as a matter of wild-domestic interface, had some rather immediate and relatively dramatic effects, such as the culling of backyard poultry on the one hand, and, on the other hand, continuation of the short lives of commercial poultry whose bodies continued their circulation, packed and labelled, in the market chain. Moreover, the sudden decrease in demand for poultry products, the restructuring of the poultry sector and official demands for stricter biosecurity measures resulted in producers incurring extra costs.[79] Thus, the biosecurity measures enforced in the name of avian influenza prevention, justified by the manner in which bio*in*security as well as biosecurity were enacted, influenced the power relations among the poultry producers. Again, this illustrates how the ordering of bio(*in*)security had far reaching effects, be-

77 Hinchliffe, Steve and Nick Bingham 2008b: 1543, the last part of this quote refers to Rabinow, Paul and Nicolas Rose 2006:197

78 Hinchliffe, Steve, John Allen, Stephanie Lavau, Nick Bingham and Simon Carter 2012:7, with reference to Karen Barad's (2007) use of the term "intra-actions".

79 Personal communication with Director of finances, poultry producing company, Balıkeşir 15.05.2007; Yalcin, Cengiz 2006

yond what was directly related to mobility and spread of the HPAI H5N1virus; separation and ordering of matters as bio*secure* or -*in*secure were, according to the market analysis report, affecting the structure of the whole Turkish poultry sector.

Throughout this volume, I will remain attentive to bio*in*security as well as biosecurity. While Bingham and Hinchliffe suggest that biosecurity is better thought of as biosecur*ing* in that it is about practices for making life safe, I aim to moving one step further back: I aim to examine how matters came to be enacted as secure or insecure in the first place. Moreover, engaging with bio(*in*)security as a processual and relational concept requires me to take into account the becoming of both the insecure and the secure. This provides two versions, at least, which may analytically realize the capacities of each other, they may disarticulate one another, and/or they may together contribute to realizing something new.[80]

80 Please refer to the previous chapter for a thorough discussion on these matters.

# 4. Studying strategies: Textual enactments of avian influenza

FAO and OIE, within the umbrella of the global framework for the control of transboundary animal diseases (GF-TADs), and in collaboration with WHO, have taken the initiative and developed the global strategy providing vision and goal towards diminishing the risk of avian influenza to humans and poultry. (… )

In order to effectively control the disease, countries should have a complete plan of action and the financial and human resources to implement it under the particular conditions prevailing in the country.[1]

Avian influenza is considered a "*global* threat", towards human as well as animal health.[2] Therefore, the two organisations of the United Nations,the Food and Agriculture Organisation (FAO) and the World Health Organization (WHO), together with the World Organisation for Animal Health (OIE), under the Global Framework for the Control of Transboundary Animal Diseases (GF-TADs) have prepared *A Global Strategy for Progressive Control of Highly Pathogenic Avian Influenza (HPAI).*[3] This "*global* threat" is also associated with national responsibility. The excerpt opening this chapter is literally in line with the Global Strategy, but taken from one of its national "offsprings", the *Strategy for Highly Pathogenic Avian Influenza Preparedness and Control in Turkey.*[4] The strategy documents can be seen as what Kristin Asdal calls *relational space*: the Global Strategy is a common ground for avian influenza control prepared by the FAO, the OIE and the WHO.[5] The Turkish National Strategy is closely connected to this "global", relational space. Expressing the official visions and goals of the internationally recognized institutions in charge of handling the global HPAI crisis, as well as Turkey's national approach to addressing the issue, these strategy documents are strategic places for studying how avian influenza is becoming a global and a national threat.[6]

1 Ivanov, Yanko 2007: pp 6–7. The first part of this excerpt can also be found in the Global Strategy (FAO, OIE and FAO 2005 Mai: ii; 2005 Nov.: vi) As it has been slightly rewritten to fit its new setting in the National Strategy ("this document" has been changed to "the global strategy") I have used this version of the text here.

2 FAO, OIE and WHO 2005 May; 2005 Nov

3 FAO, OIE and WHO 2005 May

4 Ivanov, Yanko 2007

5 Asdal, Kristin 2011b

6 FAO, OIE and WHO 2005 May: iii, 10, 13, 35, 44; 2005 Nov.: vii, 14, 18, 56; Ivanov, Yanko 2007: 72

This chapter focuses on the following question: What does avian influenza become when organizations in charge of human health (WHO), food and agriculture (FAO) and animal health (OIE) agree upon a common understanding of a global problem, a common understanding which must be considered a precondition for formulating a common strategy? Alternatively, to phrase the question in accordance with analytical approaches from science and technology studies (STS): how is avian influenza ordered and textually enacted in the Global Strategy?[7] These ways of enacting avian influenza may be seen as ways of making avian influenza real through the texts. Hence, the question emerges: how are these documents *realizing* avian influenza?[8] How is avian influenza *textualized*, *realized* and in the words of Bruno Latour, made a *matter of concern* through these documents?[9] Moreover, what happens when theses global *facts* and *concerns* become national ones, with Turkey's National Strategy? The Turkish authorities followed the recommendations of the Global Strategy to develop national and regional strategies, "country by country in a coordinated manner"[10] What happens when avian influenza spreads beyond Asia, when local outbreaks multiply across continents, and reports from these outbreaks contribute with new facts and new concerns in the re-ordering of the global issue? Finally, paying careful attention to what is going on within and between these "global" and "national" documents, this chapter reflects on how to think about "global", "national" and "local".

This chapter contains analyses of three distinct strategy documents. These are: the aforementioned Turkish National Strategy, published in 2007, and the two versions of the Global Strategy, that is what I refer to as the Draft version and Final version, published in May and November 2005, respectively. My argument is that the way avian influenza is ordered has direct implications for the biosecurity regime; it has consequences for what is *made to be* in need of protection, as well as what to protect against; which lives should be secured from what – and how.

---

7 See Asdal, Kristin 2008b; Asdal, Kristin, Kjell Lars Berge, Karen Gammelgaard, Helge Jordheim, Tore Rem, Trygve Riiser-Gundersen og Johan L. Tønnesen 2008; Law, John 1994; Mol, Annemarie 2002; Moser, Ingunn 2008.

8 An introduction to Kristins Asdal's notion on how texts are making the issue real, or how textualixing is also *realizing*, is given in Chapter 2 of this book. See also Asdal, Kristin 2008a; 2011b; 2014; Asdal, Kristin, Kjell Lars Berge, Karen Gammelgaard, Helge Jordheim, Tore Rem, Trygve Riiser-Gundersen og Johan L. Tønnesen 2008.

9 Bruno Latour's "matters of facts" and "matters of concern" are introduced in the Chapter 1. Latour, Bruno 2004. See also Barad, Karen 2003; Law, John 2004b; Moser, Ingunn 2008.

10 FAO, OIE and, WHO 2005 May: 2; Nov: 2

## The textual sites for studying avian influenza in the global-national interface

In May 2005, the FAO, the OIE and the WHO launched the draft version of their first joint *Global Strategy for the Progressive Control of Highly Pathogenic Avian Influenza (HPAI).*[11] The development of this strategy, in addition to an updated version of this document, published in November of the same year, marked a step towards a closer and more stable collaboration between the three organizations. In 2008, this collaboration led to the so-called *One World, One Health* initiative.[12] Moreover, UNICEF, the World Bank and the UN System Influenza Coordinator (UNSIC) also took part in the initiative. It was the "complexities" of highly pathogenic avian influenza and other emerging infectious diseases that made these organizations see the need for a "broad multidisciplinary and multisectoral cooperation across the animal-human-ecosystems interface".[13] I will study these Global Strategy documents, both the Draft version and the Final version, and the related Turkish National Strategy, as sites for analysing how the complex, "global" nature of avian influenza is enacted.

### Developing a Global Strategy towards HPAI based on the experience from Asia and beyond

The published Draft version of the Global Strategy builds on the experiences from HPAI in Asia, and was primarily meant to advise on the on-going *prevention, control* and*eradication*[14] efforts in this region.[15] However, an expressed ambition was to also develop "similar plans for Central Asia, Africa, America

[11] The year before, the FAO sent out their *Recommendations on the Prevention, Control and Eradication of Highly Pathogenic Avian Influenza (HPAI) in Asia* (proposed with the support of the OIE) (FAO 2004 Sept.)

[12] FAO/ECTAD 2008 Nov.

[13] FAO/ECTAD 2008 Nov.: 1

[14] Referring to FAO 2004 Sept.

[15] In this way, the local experience with avian influenza the Asian region – thus also the regional experience – is part of the Global Strategy. Thinking of what we have learned from early STS laboratory studies, as I briefly introduced in the introduction of this volume, it is also reasonable to assume that the global is also in the local. That the knowledge about the outbreaks in Asia is a (temporary) result of ordering practices involving earthly substances; mud and faeces on the protective clothes, registration forms and pencils, food, drinks and resting brakes including (or not) talks, exchange of information and information. The list is endless. Importantly, I write *temporary result* as orders are never complete. (See e.g. Law, John 1994; Law, John 2001; Law, John and Annemarie Mol 2001)

and Europe".[16] It did not take long before the need for such plans proved necessary; We can only imagine the atmosphere among the responsible delegates when, already the same month as the Draft version of the Global Strategy was published, reports started to come in that the highly pathogenic avian influenza, caused by the H5N1 serotype, was detected in Northern China, Mongolia, Russia, Kazakhstan, Romania, Croatia and Turkey.[17]

When the Final version of the strategy was published in November of the same year, the document, together with the virus, had evolved; consequently, the strategy represented itself as "a strategy for HPAI control in *and beyond* Asia."[18] As the virus had expanded its geographical territory, the document also expanded in size, from 64 to 86 pages.

The two documents appear, at the first glance, to be identical, but the "compare documents" function in Adobe Acrobat Pro makes it easy to track changes and identify the places where changes occur. While the May version of the Global Strategy was a draft, it was nonetheless published; the November version is considered as "[t]he original document".[19] By exploring what I will refer to simply as the Draft and the Final version as two sites of comparable status, I will study the impact of the changes and of the non-changes in the texts. More specifically, I will analyse how recent events have been inscribed into the new document, thus how these contribute to re-enact avian influenza.

During my analysis of these two versions of the documents, the new aspects entering with the updated text has evoked too many analytical concerns to be sufficiently dealt with within one chapter. Therefore, the current chapter will mainly, but not exclusively, concentrate on the text that remains the same – which, as I will argue, does not necessarily perform the same work – in the two versions. The following chapter will pay particular attention to text in the Final version that was changed, removed or added in order to study the impact of these changes and how they contribute to re-enacting avian influenza. For now, I will only sketch out a rough picture of the two different versions of the Global Strategy in order to provide an impression of the materiality we are dealing with when engaging with these documents.[20]

---

[16] FAO, OIE and WHO 2005 May: iii; 2005 Nov.: iv

[17] The notifications referred to here are those sent from the national authorities to the OIE which are available online at: http://www.oie.int/wahis_2/public/wahid.php/Diseaseinformation/Immsummary, *read 18.07.2014*

[18] FAO, OIE and WHO 2005 Nov: vii, *emphasis added.*

[19] FAO, OIE and WHO 2005 Nov: vi

[20] Regarding the importance of the physical form of texts or the materiality of documents, see Asdal, Kristin, Kjell Lars Berge, Karen Gammelgaard, Helge Jordheim, Tore Rem, Trygve Riiser-Gundersen og Johan L.Tønnesen 2008.

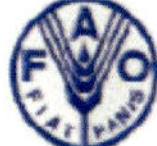

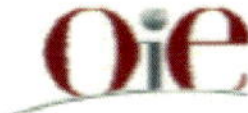


**A Global Strategy for the Progressive Control of Highly Pathogenic Avian Influenza (HPAI)**

**Food and Agriculture Organization (FAO, Rome)**
**World Organisation for Animal Health (OIE, Paris)**
**in collaboration with**
**World Health Organization (WHO, Geneva)**

**May 2005**

*The cover page of the Global Strategy Final on-line PDF version. (FAO, OIE and WHO 2005 Nov.)*

The two documents are published in Portable Document Format (PDF) and are easily accessible from the websites of the three organizations. With the exception of the relatively small colour logos of the FAO and OIE, which appear on the cover page, the entire document is in black and white, which makes it easy to print or read on the screen. While the WHO's logo is not present, text on the cover page states that the strategy was developed by the FAO and OIE "in collaboration with" the WHO. The names of individual author(s) do not appear in this document; apparently the documents have emerged out of a common understanding of these three institutions, thus carrying the authority and legitimacy these organizations possess (or not) in the global governance of infectious diseases.

Both versions of the document provide a detailed table of contents, which enables the reader to orientate his or herself within the texts easily. The documents include a list of acronyms, followed by a foreword, which is less than one page. An *Executive summary* of well five pages in the Draft version, which has expanded to ten pages in the Final version, is provided before the body text, which consists of 24 and 31 pages, respectively. This is followed by 31/44 pages back matter in the Draft- and Final version respectively, consisting of tables, figures and appendices. One appendix is newly added to the Final version, and several have been updated and extended. Obviously the map (Figure 2) displaying the "HPAI situation in Asia between 2004 and 2005" in the Draft version has been changed in the Final version, where "in Asia" was removed and it is displaying the "HPAI situation between 2004 and 2005". Thus, Appendix 6 in the Final version, which offers "Country profiles of HPAI", has also been extended. Further on, new key partners have been added to the list in Appendix 9 of the Final version, and the donor list in Appendix 5 has been extended. These are some of the major changes to the back matter of the Global Strategy documents. The final version includes a total of ten appendices; a new appendix has been added, titled "Potential risk of Highly Pathogenic Avian Influenza (HPAI) spreading through wild water bird migration".

Regarding the relationship between the body text and the back matter, the latter provides thorough and detailed information and thus supports and extends the body text, which is easy to read. References to figures, tables and appendices appear frequently in the body text, providing technical details without complicating the text. Some specificities of the relational effect within the documents, that is between the body text and the back matter, will be discussed in further detail below.

The Global Strategy recommends that regional and national plans should be carried out "country by country in a coordinated manner".[21] The Turkish National Strategy must be seen as a response to this.

## The Turkish National Strategy: Making the global issue a national concern

"The cornerstone of the national strategy is to be in compliance with the global strategy", the Turkish National Strategy states.[22] The strategy, titled *Strategy for Highly Pathogenic Avian Influenza Preparedness and Control in Turkey,* was written by international experts on behalf of the Turkish Ministry of Agriculture and Rural Affairs (MARA) as part of the so-called *Technical Assistance to Avian Influenza Preparedness & Response Project in Turkey*, here referred to as the AI project.The team who wrote the strategy document worked for the Turkish government for a two-year period in order to assist them in handling the recurring HPAI outbreaks.[23] This strategy document was written for and published with the approval of MARA's General Directorate for Protection and Control. Like in most documents produced by the project team, the front page is followed by a one-page table showing details of the project contract. Contrary to the Global Strategy, the table also provides a space for personification of the author of the national strategy, "Dr. Yanko IVANOV – Team Leader" (capital letters in original). However, the layout, colours and the use of flags and logos on the cover page clearly indicate that this document has been written within the context of a broader program. The blue/yellow European Union (EU) colours, the view from above the EU stars, down on the fragile national borders of the European counties, and, at the bottom, the flags of both the EU and Turkey, MARA's emblem, can be seen as adding authority and legitimacy to this document. It is outside the scope of my work to evaluate the effect of this symbolism. However, the comments made, by the Turkish

21 FAO, OIE and WHO 2005 May: 2; 2005 Nov: 2

22 Ivanov, Yanko 2007:72

23 As of 18 July 2014, the English part of the project website was still available at: http://www.prwatson.co.uk/TR_06_AI_SV/English/start.htm. In addition to developing an avian influenza strategy and improving the regulatory framework, the project group was assigned a wide range of tasks. For example, these were related to education and training, addressing poultry industry problems, proposing ways of improving biosecurity in backyard poultry, improving laboratory diagnostic capabilities, strengthening preparedness and response capabilities, upgrading veterinary information systems, and assessing and carrying out epidemiological studies and surveillance programmes. Chapter 6 of this book will analyse how the outbreak investigations, which became another central task for the AIproject, contributed to enacting avian influenza in very particular ways.

farmers, which I refer to in my introduction, remind us not to take the legitimacy of international authorities for granted. I am specifically referring to the comment made by the neighbour of an outbreak farm who referred to avian influenza as a "*komplot*" supported by the EU.[24]

Like all public documents produced by the project, this strategy has been published on the project website and on the website of MARA in both English and Turkish. I primarily work with the English versions, and for the purpose of my reading and analysis, it is useful to work with the electronic version of the document. Despite the colourful cover page, the aforementioned table that is also in colour, and headings and sub headings in blue, green and brown, also this document is easy to print. However, a hard copy of the document was given to individuals considered important for avian influenza prevention and response during various workshops and training exercises around the country.[25] Workshop and training participants included national, provincial and local authorities, veterinaries, health personnel and representatives from the poultry sector.

In March 2007, a few months before the National Strategy was published, the FAO, the OIE and the WHO publish a fully revised Global Strategy. One could therefore assume that the global strategy document referred to here is this 2007 version. As major parts of the text in the National Strategy are identical to the 2005 Global Strategy, in particular to the Final version published in November, it must however, be the global strategy document published already in 2005 that the National Strategy associates with. This close relationship between the documents provides an opportunity to study what happens with the text when it is moved from the general and global to the more specific national setting.[26]

The National Strategy consists of 84 pages, 6 of which are front matter, such as cover pages, tables, a detailed table of contents and a list of abbre-

24 During my fieldwork in 2007, I heard many other similar comments. Often the mistrust was also directed towards the national authorities as people refused to acknowledge the importance or existence of avian influenza; people would tell me that it was something from Ankara, meaning that it was not a real disease, but a political intervention ordered by national authorities. See also: Durutan, Nedret and Okan Cünyet 2006; n.d.; Geerlings, Ellen 2006

25 AIproject Progress report 7, November 2008 http://www.prwatson.co.uk/TR_06_AI_SV/English/start.htm, *last read 21.10.13*

26 In addition to the global text, content from an Africa-based strategy also found its way into the Turkish National Strategy. After some research, it became apparent that several parts of the text were also identical to the African strategy. As the latter was published before the Turkish National Strategy, it is reasonable to assume that the text was taken from the Africa based strategy (FAO/ECTAD 2007)

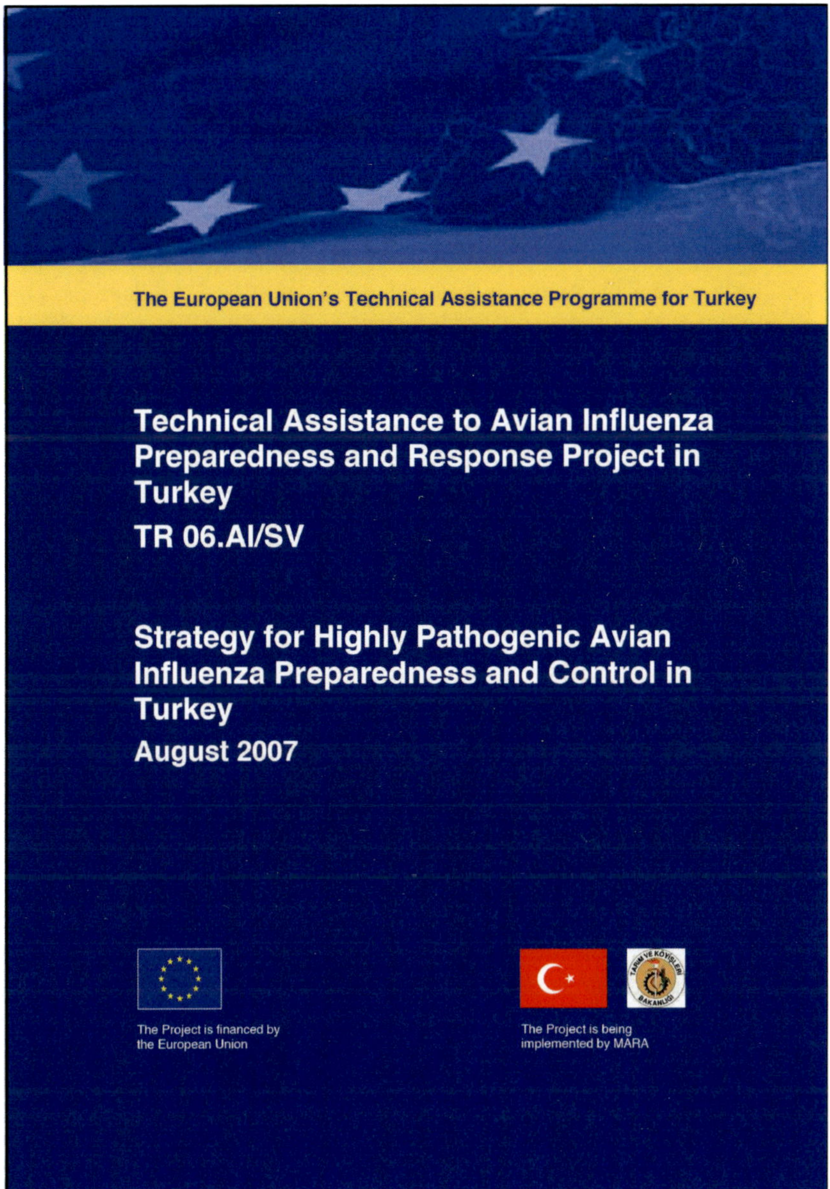


*The cover page of the on-line PDF version of the Turkish National Strategy. (Ivanov, Yanko 2007)*

viations. The body text starts with a one-page introduction, followed by a three page executive summary and a "Global AI [avian influenza] situation assessment" which is less than a page long.[27] The assessment of the avian influenza situation in Turkey comprises 29 pages. The section titled Strategy is four pages long. Two longer sections follow: an overview of "Tools and Methods Available for Control of AI in Turkey" (22 pages) and "Constraints and Challenges to HPAI Control" (20 pages). In addition, the report includes the following sections: "Implementation" (six pages), "Technical and Policy Considerations for the National Strategy" (one page), and "Reduce the Opportunity for Human Infection" (one page). Two pages is lining out "Strategic Research to Guide Control Measures" before the National Strategy rounds off with a short sections (less than one page) on "Applied Research", "Outputs", and "Impacts". With the exception of the assessments of the global and national avian influenza situation, the majority of the text is copied directly from the Global Strategy with minimal changes, such as reference to "global" which has turned into "national".-

## Choosing versions to hold on

There are several reasons why I have chosen to focus on the first global strategy and its Turkish national companion, rather than later versions of the strategy documents.[28] A main reason relates to timing. These are the strategies that were operative during the years when outbreaks were reported in Turkey, a period that coincided with my field trips. By focussing on these versions, I remain close to the material I will work with in the following chapters. The Global Strategy was already published when I began my project, but the Turkish National Strategy was in the process of being written when I visited AVIAN INFLUENZA project's office in Ankara during my first fieldtrip. As previously mentioned, there are direct links between this Global Strategy and the Turkish National Strategy in that large pieces of text have been copied from the first and passed on to the latter. Therefore, a central concern of this chapter is to examine the impact of this re-placement; how does text change when it moves

[27] Ivanov, Yanko 2007: 11

[28] Another document which I studied in-depth during the early phase of my research was *FAO Recommendations on the Prevention, Control, and Eradication of Highly Pathogenic Avian Influenza (HPAI) in Asia*, published in September 2004. This so called position paper can be seen as a predecessor to the Global Strategy that would appear in 2005, which was a result of cooperation between the FAO, the OIE and the WHO. The Global Strategy was revised and published by the three organizations; the Turkish National Strategy has also been revised

to, and works from, a new place, and how does the text contribute in enacting its new surroundings?

Regarding the Global Strategy, a second reason for choosing to focus on the 2005 edition is that its two versions, the draft and the final document, provide an excellent opportunity to witness how the strategy documents changed with the development of the epidemic.[29] These documents make it possible to study how avian influenza has been textualized and made real in these documents, and how the manner in which avian influenza was made to matter in the first place contributed to the re-ordering of the "global threat" as the virus spread from Asia to Europe. The initial avian influenza outbreak reported in Turkey are among those experiences that were taken into account, referred to and put to work in the Final version of the Global Strategy. By following some of the experiences that are brought into the Global Strategy, for example via outbreak reports, I aim to see how "local experiences" are translated into the "global setting". Some aspects related to the spread and the inscription of this in the Final version, will be studied even further in the next chapter; the current and the following chapter aim to explore how the avian influenza spreading to Europe is inscribed in these strategy documents; the chapters will examine how local outbreaks contribute to the ordering and re-ordering of the "global threat" of avian influenza.

## Exploring the heterogeneities of avian influenza

*Looking down* at the strategies,[30] I will now *go close to the object*, avian influenza, and explore how avian influenza is enacted in these documents.[31] Is it

---

29 The Foreword of the Global Strategy (Final version) states that "[s]ince the inception of this document in May 2005, avian influenza has *progressed* (...) well beyond the originally infected foci in Southeast and East Asia. The toll in human fatalities and cases has continued to rise, with increasing concerns that the final evolution of the disease, namely human-to-human transfer of HPAI, may trigger a pandemic." (FAO, OIE; WHO 2005 Oct: vi, italics added).

30 I am here putting Law's (2004:19) Leibniz inspired strategy of looking down for "complexity in the detail" rather than "up for 'the broader picture'".(See also the introduction and the introduction to this chapter.)

31 I am particularly drawing on Asdal (2014) here. Asdal stresses, "that we need to get closer to the object". This time, her object is milk, and she is showing "how the object 'mother's milk' was enacted as 'natural' [by taking] other, and related, versions of milk into account." In order to do so she is studying how milk was enacted different through different relations; "within (...) different versions of medicine" and "within a version of the economy: the free market economy". These different versions are coming together in a "*relational space*" where the mothers' milk is enacted as natural. Asdal is further developing her concept of the

so that we can find, in these documents, a common understanding and a clear agreement on "the avian influenza crisis", to paraphrase the title of the Global Strategy? Do the strategy documents provide an answer to what avian influenza *is* and how to handle it? Or, thinking for example of the various answers to my question at the beginning of this volume, do these strategy documents provide space for various versions of avian influenza? And if so, what implications does this have for *control*, which is the word used in the title of both the Turkish National Strategy and the Global Strategy? In order to study this, I will now analyse how avian influenza has been enacted as four heterogeneous avian influenza issues in these three related strategy documents.

### An emerging disease issue

Over the last several decades, an average of one *newly emerging disease* per year has been identified, of which 75% have been of the zoonotic type. Their transboundary nature highlights that no country can count itself exempt from such diseases.[32]

The text quoted here is one of several places in the Global Strategy where avian influenza is enacted as an emerging disease issue. Emerging diseases, in this text, represent a threat to *all countries*; the "transboundary nature" of emerging diseases, as mentioned in this excerpt, works to legitimize a Global Strategy. No clear definition of 'emerging diseases' appears in the strategy documents. However, in other places the WHO states than an emerging disease is one "that has appeared in a population for the first time, or that may have existed previously but is rapidly increasing in incidence or geographic range."[33] This definition is twofold; it is about *emergence as origin,* and *emergence as geographical spread*. Do these versions of emergence also appear in

"relational space", as mentioned in a previous article, in this book. (Asdal, Kristin 2011b).

32 FAO, OIE and WHO 2005 May: 1; 2005Nov: 1, *italics added.* (This text is not included in the National Strategy) (Ivano, Yankovic 2007).

33 http://www.who.int/topics/emerging_diseases/en/, read 29.07.2014. The OIE provides a slightly more technical definition on their website: "An emerging disease is defined as a new infection resulting from the evolution or change of an existing pathogen or parasite resulting in a change of host range, vector, pathogenicity or strain; or the occurrence of a previously unrecognised infection or disease." (http://www.oie.int/for-the-media/editorials /detail/article/emerging-and-re-emerging-zoonoses/) In the *Report of the WHO/FAO/OIE joint consultation on emerging zoonotic diseases* held in Geneva, Switzerland 3.-5. May 2004 (FAO; WHO and OIE 2004: ) it is states that "[t]the participants agreed on the following definition of an emerging zoonosis: An emerging zoonosis is a zoonosis that is newly recognized or newly evolved, or that has occurred previously but shows an increase in incidence or expansion in geographical, host or vector range."

the strategies? A closer look makes it apparent that indeed they do, however, the interesting thing is to examine how they work; how do they contribute to enacting avian influenza as an emerging disease issue?

## Emergence as origin: A matter of back matter

Detailed descriptions of the "evolution" of "Highly Pathogenic Avian influenza (HPAI), also known as fowl plague, [which] is a disease of birds causing huge morbidity and mortality", appears in Appendix 2 of the Global Strategy.This appendix, titled "HPAI Virus in Asia: Technical Information", provides technical information on how the HPAI virus evolves genetically *from* the low pathogenic avian influenza (LPAI) virus. This technical information builds on "available evidence" that associates "benign" LPAI with wildlife, and HPAI with domestic poultry:

> While the gene pool of the avian influenza viruses is relatively benign in its natural wildlife population hosts, it can evolve rapidly *into pathogenic strains* after infecting and adapting to domestic poultry. Available evidence points towards factors such as the changing population size and structure of the poultry industry *in response to increasing consumer demand*, the expansion of virus circulation from its traditional host range to domestic ducks and terrestrial poultry, and its wide geographical spread through trade in live birds being the main reasons for concern.[34]

This general origin story has also been transferred, almost word for word, directly to the body text of the strategy document, and later to the Turkish National Strategy. However, two details have been lost along the way, as indicated by text in italics in the excerpt above, and one is added. First, while the appendix states that "the [benign] avian influenza virus ( . . . ) can evolve rapidly *into pathogenic strains* after infecting and adapting to domestic poultry", the body text states only that the virus "can evolve rapidly [text removed!] after infecting and adapting to domestic poultry."[35] Removing the specificity, "into pathogenic strain", when the text moves into the body text, also removes the crucial point; that it is in the meeting with domestic poultry that the virus might gain its lethal powers. The role of domestic poultry in the evolvement of HPAI becomes blurred as the text moves (and some of it does not move) from the appendix to the body text.

---

34 FAO, OIE and WHO 2005 May: 3; 2005 Nov: 3 and 48 (Appendix2); Ivanov, Yanko 2007: 77, *italics added.*

35 FAO, OIE and WHO 2005 May: 3 and Appendix 2; 2005 Nov: 3 and Appendix 2; Ivanov, Yanko 2007: 77

The second detail that gets lost on the way from appendix to body text of the Global Strategy, and which is also not present when this section is moved further to the Turkish National Strategy, is the connection that is made, in the appendix, between emergence and "increasing consumer demands". Like the appendix, the body text states, "the main reasons for concern" are the "[a]vailable [pieces of ] evidence [which] points towards factors such as the changing population size and structure of the poultry industry" and so on. However, while the appendix establishes a direct relationship and sees the changes in the poultry production as something that happens "in response to increasing consumer demand," this latter part of the sentence is not to be found in the body text. Consequently, in the body text of the strategies, consumers are not placed in relation to the *emergence* of HPAI at all; any causal relationship between consumer demands and the "HPAI crisis" are left behind; they remain in the appendix – in the back matter of the Global Strategy. "Available evidence", or these current *matters of fact* as Latour would say,are given the status as "main reasons for concern" in the appendix, or in the back matter, of the Global Strategy. However, they are not made to matter in the body text. This shows how facts are only partially finding their way to the inline texts, and the effects thereof: As text moves from the back matter to the body text, concerns related to emergence become less of a matter regarding domestic poultry and consumer demands, and more of a matter relating to wildlife.

There are also other incidents of re-ordering of technical or virological events as they move from the back matter to the body text of the Global Strategy. In the body text of both the Global Strategy and the Turkish National Strategy, a list of so-called "rationale" and "key reasons" for the strategy clarifies a number of issues. Among these that:

- HPAI results from low pathogenic avian influenza (LPAI), which is present in wild birds in many parts of the world.[36]

This is the only place in the body text of the Global Strategy that explicitly mentions LPAI. Similar to the technical information in the appendix, LPAI is here put in relation to wild birds. However, unlike the appendix, this bullet pointed sentence does not touch upon the processes or the conditions that enable LPAI to *result* in HPAI. Simplifications and generalizations contribute to downplaying potential controversies and make the facts more applicable to other settings.

[36] FAO, OIE and WHO 2005 May: 3,*bold letters only in original*; Nov: 3, *bold letters only in original*; Ivanov, Yanko 2007: 8, *no bold letters in original*

The Turkish National Strategy differs slightly from the Global Strategy in the way it treats the technical or virological events that may enable HPAI viruses to evolve. In the Turkish National Strategy, the following "rationale", directly related to emergence, is added to this list:

- Low pathogenic AI strains should also be considered because AI virus show a continuous spectrum of pathogenicity in gallinaceous poultry, from no pathogenicity to high pathogenicity and LPAI (H5 or H7) virus can mutate into an HPAI virus.[37]

In contrast to the Global Strategy, the Turkish National Strategy explicitly advocates "specific surveillance systems to detect infection with LPAI as soon as it appears" as well as "a timely assessment of whether there has been spread *to* the industrial poultry population in the area".[38] The strategy does not only call for surveillance, assessment as well as reporting of LPAI and HPAI; it also recommends that "[c]ompensation payments should also be considered in case of culling flocks infected with LPAI strains because the virus can mutate into an HPAI virus (. . . )".[39] Even though this is not a concern that receives much attention in the Turkish National Strategy, this document does highlight that domestic poultry is an environment in which LPAI viruses can turn highly pathogenic; moreover, it offers relatively detailed recommendations regarding how this can be prevented.

What should be noticed is that, with the exception of the one aforementioned bullet pointed sentence, the body text of the Global Strategy is exclusively concerned with HPAI; it is "[t]he *HPAI* viruses [that] are of particular concern".This observation makes me realize that I have probably gone down the wrong track in terms of exploring what the strategies say about the *emergence* of *emerging* diseases or even the emergence of HPAI.

Regarding the strategies, the matter of concern is not *emergence* in the sense of *originating*. Rather, they are concerned about an *ongoing crisis*. The focus of these documents is *not about preventing emergence* but about preventing (further) *spread;*[40] it is about preventing *transmission,*[41] preventing (fur-

[37] Ivanov, Yanko 2007: 8. The importance of "LPAI monitoring" is also stressed other places in the National Strategy, e.g. at the very beginning of the chapter titled *Constraints and Challenges to HPAI Control,* where the rest of the text of the introductory section is identical to the Global Strategy but the National Strategy adds that "[s]pecial attention needs also to be paid to LPAI monitoring( . . . )" (p57)

[38] Ivanov, Yanko 2005:31, *italics added.*

[39] Ivanov, Yanko 2005: 45

[40] FAO, OIE AND WHO 2005 Nov: vii, viii, ix, 5, 11; Ivanov, Yanko 2007: 9, 13, 29, 57, 58, 59, 62.

[41] Ivanov, Yanko 2007: 40, 64 (transmission).

ther) *introduction,*[42] preventing *incursion,*[43] preventing the disease from *taking hold,*[44] preventing *creation of endemic areas,*[45] preventing *recurrence,*[46] and preventing *risk to human health.*[47] By studying the appendix, I was able trace how emergence is understood. While a direct relation between poultry rearing practices and emergence, as origin, of highly pathogenic avian influenza viruses are working as a matter of fact in the appendices, this is not the matter of concern in the body text of the Global Strategy, and only of minimal concern in the National Strategy. The theories of emergence as origin that are at work in the appendix are not challenged in the body text of the Global Strategy. They are simply of no concern.

## Emergence as spread: New places, different relations, joining the category of emerging infectious transboundary zoonotic diseases

Realizing that avian influenza as an emerging disease in these strategy documents is *not* about origin but about *spread* also highlights the actuality of the terms *transboundary* and *zoonotic* that are often added, making avian influenza an *emerging transboundary zoonotic disease.* This label draws together diseases due to their ability to spread, including across geographical borders (transboundary), and move between species (zoonotic). As an *emerging transboundary zoonotic disease*, avian influenza is associated with other serious diseases, such as "bovine spongiform encephalopathy (BSE, mad cow disease) Nipah virus [and] Severe Acute Respiratory Syndrome (SARS)".[48] The "*transboundary nature*" of these diseases make them fit into the even broader category of transboundary animal diseases (TADs), where they are associated with more threatening diseases such as "e.g. foot and mouth disease (FMD) and

[42] FAO, OIE AND WHO 2005 Nov: ix, 5, 19, 20, 27; Ivanov, Yanko 2007: 8, 9, 16, 40, 62 (introduction).

[43] FAO, OIE and WHO 2005 Nov: 10 (incursion).

[44] FAO, OIE and WHO 2005 Nov: viii (taking hold).

[45] FAO, OIE and WHO 2005 Nov: 20; Ivanov, Yanko 2007: 10 (endemic).

[46] FAO, OIE and WHO 2005 Nov: 17; Ivanov, Yanko 2007: 40 (recurrence).

[47] FAO, OIE and WHO 2005 Nov: 3, 20, 29; Ivanov, Yanko 2007: 8 (human health). Both the Global Strategy and the Turkish National Strategy frequently mention prevention in very general terms such as 'preparedness and prevention strategies', 'preventive measures' or 'measures for prevention and control' (FAO, OIE and WHO 2005 Nov: 16, 20, 24, 30, 20, 29; Ivanov, Yanko 2007: 6, 11, 14, 16, 21, 30, 31, 34, 35, 37, 38, 54, 55, 57, 63). Most of the time they do not specify what this involves and they do not appear to directly or indirectly refer to 'prevent(ing)' the emergence (in the sense of originating) of HPAI.

[48] FAO, OIE and WHO 2005 Nov: 1

classical swine fever (CSF)".[49] Leaving out emerging and using animal rather than zoonotic, this concept is broader, covering diseases in animals (without considering possible human-animal transmission) that may cross national borders.[50]

What are the effects of this categorization? What implications does categorization have on how avian influenza is enacted as an emerging disease issue? First of all, I will argue, when the issue of emergence is getting less a matter of origin and nearly exclusively a matter of spread, it is also the latter that the strategies aim to, according to their titles, "control"; this is a strategy aiming to control spread of something that has already originated, HPAI H5N1. It is not a strategy to prevent LPAI to turn HPAI. Furthermore, categorization works to make avian influenza part of larger and growing, a worldwide concern. Categorization contributes to removing the extraordinary and the exceptional with regards to the specific HPAI caused by the H5N1 virus. Rather than being exceptional, the virus becomes one among many diseases covered by these categories. Avian influenza becomes normalized; it is about *normalization* as avian influenza becomes one of many diseases which most of us have heard of. Moreover, it becomes a normal, a "natural", part of the disease ecology of modern animal trade.

Recalling the text I borrowed from the Global Strategy when introducing avian influenza as an emerging disease issue above, "[o]ver the last several decades an average of one newly emerging disease per year has been identified (... ). Their transboundary nature highlights that no country can count itself exempt from such diseases."[51] Emergence of new diseases – and avian influenza is among them – is, in the strategies, made common; such diseases are, in this strategy, *normal, everywhere.* A parallel can be drawn to Asdal's study that shows how air pollution was normalized; how it was made an ordinary and normal, "*allment og alminnelig*", part of industrialization. In the Norwegian context, Asdal studies how the phenomenon "local smoke damages" became a sub-phenomenon of a more general phenomenon that was taking place in industrialized countries, whose level of development was comparable

49 FAO, OIE and WHO 2005 Nov: 1; "Global threat" is frequently used in the Global Strategy with reference to HPAI (FAO, OIE and WHO 2005 May: iii, 4, 29, 55; 2005 Nov: vii, 4, 39, 69.)

50 According to the FAO and OIE, "Transboundary animal diseases are defined as: those that are of significant economic, trade and/or food security importance for a considerable number of countries; which can easily spread to other countries and reach epidemic proportions; and where control/management, including exclusion, requires cooperation between several countries." (FAO and OIE 2004 May)

51 FAO, OIE and WHO 2005 May: 1; 2005 Nov: 1

with Norway; it was *normalized*. Similarly, I will argue, in the strategy documents studied here, the emergence of transboundary animal diseases are also being normalized; according to the Global Strategy, such diseases ought to be expected in a globalized world. Similarly, Doreen Massey writes about "globalisation *in this particular form* which is ( . . . ) taken as being inevitable".[52] Normalizing air pollution and newly emerging transboundary diseases is also about making it what Massey critically refers to as a "self-evident truth" that such side effects become "inevitable"; co-producing such side effects are made an unquestioned and integral part of development.[53]

The third and closely related implication of this categorization is that turning avian influenza into a transboundary animal disease, or a TAD, draws a particular connection beyond the virus-host relation. Consulting the FAO and OIE's definition, TADs or "[t]ransboundary animal diseases[,] are defined as: those that are of significant economic, trade and/or food security importance for a considerable number of countries (. . . )".[54] In this way, avian influenza, as an emerging disease issue, becomes a matter of "global" economy.[55] Hence, by studying avian influenza as an emerging disease issue, another issue emerges and calls for attention. That is, avian influenza as an economic issue.

## An economic issue

"Why a global strategy?" This question is opening the *Executive summary* of the Global Strategy, and the answer is immediately given: "The continuing outbreaks of highly pathogenic avian influenza (HPAI) ( . . . ) have been disastrous to the poultry industry in the region and have raised serious global public health concerns."[56] The extent of the economic impact of HPAI is further emphasised. For example, in both versions of the Global Strategy a section is devoted to this issue:

2.8 Economic impact and poultry trade are in jeopardy

Over 150 million poultry were destroyed as the result of the 2003 and 2004 HPAI outbreaks in Asia. The direct and indirect economic impact, while still being evaluated, has reached millions of dollars. Trade in poultry at the domestic, regional and

---

52 Massey, Doreen 2005: 83

53 Massey, Doreen 2005: 84

54 FAO and OIE 2004 May

55 Again, it worth noting that the global is something that is locally embedded; in this instance, it is evident through certain processes within and between the FAO and the OIE that lead to the development of the "Global Framework for Transboundary Animal Diseases"

56 FAO, OIE and WHO 2005 May: iii; 2005 Nov: vii

international levels has been severely affected. The total losses in GDP accruing from the damaged poultry sector in Asia amounted to $10 billion. If the direct health risk impact from avian influenza in birds is added to the overall negative impact problem on livestock and the drop in tourism, economic losses would be considerably higher ( ... ).[57]

A full overview of the economic costs associated with avian influenza were not available at the time of writing the Global Strategy, both because new outbreaks were still being detected (this was still the case at the time of finalizing this book) and because of the complexities of accounting the direct and indirect costs. Nonetheless, preliminary estimates establish avian influenza as an economic issue with severe impacts. The Global Strategy also draws on data from previous outbreaks of other diseases to emphasise the extent of avian influenza as a "world-wide" economic issue: "While the economic losses from TADs ( ... ), in Europe have been well documented, it is the newly emerging zoonotic diseases that are causing increasing world-wide concern."[58]

By enacting avian influenza as an economic issue, the Global Strategy contributes to establish the disease as an immense issue; it is "world-wide" concern, and the numbers appear high. Nikolas Rose has shown how numbers are a key condition for present forms of government because they help to produce the very object. Furthermore, Asdal has shown how "numerical technologies not only describe already existing realities, but also help to produce these realities in the first place."[59] But, what realities emerge when we pay closer attention to avian influenza as an economic issue?[60] How do these realities implicate avian influenza "*control*", a term used in the headings of the strategy documents? What needs to be *controlled* when avian influenza is enacted as a heterogeneous economic issue?

## The economy: A victim in need of protection

In the Global Strategy, avian influenza is immediately introduced as something that has negative economic impacts across social classes, on various production systems and beyond national borders. The document also states that it may hamper opportunities for positive economic development. For example, the economy is enacted as a victim of avian influenza in the Executive Summary:

57 FAO, OIE and WHO 2005 May: iii; 2005 Nov: vii

58 FAO, OIE and WHO 2005 May: 1; 2005 Nov: 1

59 Asdal, Kristin 2007: 311, with reference to Nikolas Rose (1999: 198)

60 In a thorough study which poses related questions (but considers other empirical material), Asdal explores how "theories and practices of economics and accounting contribute" to how "[n]ature-wholes emerge, are enacted, and take part in politics" (Asdal; Kristin 2008a: 123).

[HPAI] is causing (... ) economic losses and threatening the livelihood of hundreds of millions of poor livestock farmers, jeopardizing smallholder entrepreneurship and commercial poultry production and seriously impeding regional and international trade and market opportunities.[61]

Avian influenza is negatively affecting the economy of the poor as well as international trade relations. Within the Introduction, avian influenza is enacted as a direct threat to economic development:

There are substantial opportunities for economic growth, particular in rural areas, to be fuelled by this process, widely termed "Livestock Revolution". However, these opportunities are being threatened by emerging transboundary animal diseases, many of which are zoonotic in nature. Therefore the control of such *trade-limiting diseases* is becoming ever more important.[62]

Interestingly, transboundary animal diseases are renamed as "trade-limiting diseases". In the previous section, HPAI became part of this larger category of transboundary animal diseases; consequently, it became normalized, and the critical point was spread rather than origin. Now, this group of diseases have been made responsible for hindering a "Livestock Revolution", which here, in the body text of the Global Strategy, stands for something exclusively positive, that is "substantial opportunities for economic growth".[63] This exclusive positivity to a "Livestock Revolution" in the body text, depends on leaving behind concerns in the appendix related to the negative side-effects of such a revolution, such as the *origin* of new and the re-emergence of diseases.

Moving on to the Turkish National Strategy, the economic threat of HPAI is among the "key reasons" and "rationale for developing and implementing a national strategy":

- The poultry sector in Turkey is an important agriculture sector. The commercial sector's annual turnover is about US$ 3 billion, making it one of the most developed agricultural/ industrial sectors in Turkey. The AI threat therefore has important economic and social implications.[64]

---

61 FAO, OIE and WHO 2005 Nov: vii

62 FAO, OIE and WHO 2005 May: 1; 2005 Nov: 1, *italics added.*

63 Ibid. Transboundary animal diseases also cause negative impacts on tourism. The outbreak of Severe Acute Respiratory Syndrome (SARS) in 2003 illustrates that this is a threat. SARS that affected "several hundred people in large parts of South international and Southeast Asia and Canada" Furthermore, "[i]nternational travel and tourism were severely curtailed by the outbreak of SARS in Asia. The disease took over a year to be brought under control (... )" (FAO, OIE and WHO 2005May: 1; 2005Nov: 1).

64 Ivanov, Yanko 2007: 8. This same sentence can also be found in point 4.4: *Poultry production sector profile* on p. 23. In the section above, I mentioned that the Turkish National

Like most other places, the strategy does not here either show explicitly *how* "AI" is a "threat". How does a virus "infect" and affect the economy? The Turkish National Strategy provides a few specific examples that add nuances to the relations between HPAI and economic impacts: "[m]ass depopulation [due to culling]( … ) has recently given rise to high costs and economical losses for governments, stakeholders and, ultimately, for consumers."[65] Furthermore, the strategy emphasises that "[n]ew destinations have to be found for spent hens, which were formerly sold to backyard poultry farmers. This trade is now forbidden, resulting in heavy economic losses for egg producers."[66] As mentioned in the introduction of this book, in the case of Turkey, spent hens primarily refers to egg producing hens, or layer hens, thus "spent layers", from commercial enterprises that, due to age or other factors, no longer meet the productivity demands of the commercial egg producers. These hens are sold directly from cars or at markets to so-called backyard poultry holders, where they continue their life as "retired", commonly among 6 to 60 other backyard poultry, or *köy tavuk*, literally "village hen". By paying attention to "mass depopulation" and banning the sale of spent hens, the Turkish National Strategy is distributing the responsibility for the negative economic impacts onto the measures implemented to combat the disease. It is not (only) the virus itself, but rather the disease control and eradication measures that cause negative economic impacts.

Spent hens are interesting in that they are a bridge between the formal, commercial poultry sector and the informal backyard poultry across the country. The spent hens market in Turkey is vast, and involves an intricate and unregistered network of private spent hen retailers, which distribute birds from commercial integrations, primarily located in north-western parts of the country, to backyard poultry holders all over the country, particularly in the east.[67] The reason for prohibiting the sale of spent hens is not explicitly mentioned in the Turkish National Strategy, however, according to studies on impacts of avian influenza in Turkey published by others, the law came as a direct consequence of the early, countrywide wave of HPAI spread, and was quickly im-

Strategy added LPAI (in relation to possible emergence of HPAI) to the list of key rationales for an AI strategy, which is basically identical to the list of key reasons stated in the Global Strategy. The second and final change is the inclusion of the country specific rationale.

65 Ivanov, Yanko 2007: 59, 78. Here it is also mentioned that the "slaughter and destruction of large numbers of animals is also questionable from an ethical point of view, particularly when the human health implications are negligible."

66 Ivanov, Yanko 2007: 23

67 Geerlings, Ellen 2006; Durutan, Nedret and Okan, Cüneyt 2006

plemented due to the high risk of disease spread involved in this activity.[68] As the possible involvement of the distribution of spent hens in the spread of avian influenza is *not explicitly* mentioned in the Turkish National Strategy,this specific activity, like the formal sector in general, is enacted as victim of HPAI – *not* as a possible cause.

In my explorations of the Global Strategy and the Turkish National Strategy, I have now traced how avian influenza is harmful *to* the economy, both directly and indirectly. The following bullet pointed sentence on the list of "key reasons", or rationale, for both the Turkish National Strategy and the Global Strategy, works to underscore this:

- HPAI threatens regional and international trade and places the global poultry industry in the developed and developing worlds at risk.[69]

Even though the texts do not explicitly explain *how* HPAI represent a threat, the text above clearly states the relationship and the *direction* of influence between the disease and the economy; the economy is the *victim* of transboundary animal diseases in general, and HPAI in particular, and *has to be protected.* However, the direction of influence may also veer in the opposite direction.

### The economy: A cause that has to be controlled

- HPAI has emerged and spread rapidly *as a consequence of* globalized markets.[70]

This statement also appears in the key rationale for both for the Global Strategy and the Turkish National strategy. Hence, it is not only the viruses and the measures against them that cause economic loss; bluntly, one can say that the strategy documents are depicting this as a chicken/egg relationship as the factors related to economic activity are pointed out as propelling the spread of the disease. This is made quite clear in the Global Strategy:

With a large and growing volume of regional and international trade in livestock and livestock products and the rapid movement of large numbers of people across continents through air travel, several emerging infectious zoonotic diseases are spreading widely and quickly over large geographical regions.[71]

In this way, the Global Strategy is enacting economic activity and humanly induced mechanisms as a cause for the spread of the disease.

68 *Ibid*

69 FAO, OIE and WHO 2005 May: 2; 2005 Nov: 2; Ivanov, Yanko 2007: 8

70 *Op. cit., italics added.*

71 FAO, OIE and WHO 2005 May: 1; 2005 Nov:1

Also, the Turkish National Strategy discusses the spread of HPAI in relation to economic and commercial activities. More specifically, the strategy states that the "*[i]nformal* domestic poultry trade within the country may also [in addition to "potential contact with migratory birds"] contribute to the dispersal or spread of HPAI."[72] By explicitly and exclusively making this an issue about *informal* trade, the Turkish National Strategy is, with this sentence, establishing a border between the formal and informal poultry sector; a border that in practice is much more vague.[73] This border works to make this an issue of *informal* poultry trade, exclusively. Hence, in this instance, the Turkish National Strategy is not including the formal domestic poultry sector; the formal sector is kept out when the economic activities are is enacted as a cause for the problems.

However, there is one aspect of the text where the Turkish National Strategy does recognize the possibility of a relationship between commercial poultry trade and avian influenza. While this relationship is not explicitly stated, it is reasonable to assume that this concerns both formal and informal trade:

> Commercial poultry trade along the Istanbul – Ankara – Anatolia routes might have been involved in AI spread, with many trucks travelling through potentially infected areas, increasing the risk of disease transmission. Daily close contact with backyard poultry and poor biosecurity helped the disease to spread rapidly.[74]

An interesting twist is taking place in this text; initially it states that "[c]ommercial poultry trade (… ) might have been involved in AI spread". However, it is the "potentially infected areas" on the way that may have *added* virus to the trucks. Any possibility for a HPAI infectious agent to depart from the holdings where "[c]ommercial poultry" were loaded on the trucks is here being distributed to "potentially infected areas" along the way where "many trucks [were] travelling through". Commercial trade may have been "involved"

72 Ivanov, Yanko 2007: 65, *italics added.*

73 The fact that many contracting farmers have their own backyard poultry in their garden, adjacent to the coops where they grow broilers for contracting companies is one example of the fragile border between the formal and informal sector. The vast spent hens market in Turkey, which involves an intricate and undocumented network of private spent hens retailers distributing birds from commercial integrations to backyard poultry holders all over the country, is another example highlighting the usefulness of attending to borderlands, rather than fixed, clear borders (jfr. Hinchliffe, Steve, John Allen, Stephanie Lavau, Nick Bingham and Simon Carter 2012:)Neither the Global Strategy nor the Turkish National Strategy reflects on the blurred distinction between the formal and informal trade of poultry or poultry products.

74 Ivanov, Yanko 2007: 23

in spreading AI *further*, however, no opening is given for critical inquiry of the place where the original load, "commercial poultry", originated from.

In relation to their study of avian influenza in the United Kingdom, Steve Hinchliffe et al. argue that the concern of the spread of disease entails "a particular geographical imagination wherein an increasingly networked planet enhances disease spread".[75] The "commercial poultry trade along the Istanbul – Ankara – Anatolia routes" as stated in the Turkish National Strategy, may be said to represent such a network for disease spread. With reference to Stephen S. Morse Hinchliffe et al. argue that the "contemporary direction of this 'viral traffic' is often from 'zoonotic pools' in the Global South and East, towards the North and West[76], a reversal of the pre-colonial tendency for disease to follow empire."[77] The Turkish National Strategy is reproducing a parallel dichotomy where rural villages resemble "the Global South and East" and the metropolises, Istanbul and Ankara, resemble the "North and West". Hence, I will argue, the Turkish National Strategy is reproducing what Hinchliffe et al. call a "networked disease model" where disease spread is conceived within a "geometric or topographical framework" and that it is "operating with a one way direction where pathogens enters "*into* a healthy population".[78] Hinchliffe et al. argue that it is less about *topography* and disease as a fixed unit that moves and keeps its shape within networks; rather they call for a *topological* approach to disease preparedness which offers space for the mutable nature of viral connections and which may be sensitive to the unpredictable twists of pathogens. Similarly, anthropologist Meike Wolf emphasises the need to realize and deal with the shortcomings of prediction and stringent planning when understanding and managing influenza. Wolf stresses the importance of making space for flexibility and change as well as interconnections. "Recognition of the linkage of other organisms and other places to the human body", Wolf writes, "suggests that there is a need for a biocultural reconception of influenza and its impact on our understanding of the topology of the body."[79] If the Turkish National Strategy exercised a topological approach, the direction of spread would have been kept open and possible in two ways; the trucks would not

75 Hinchliffe, Steve, John Allen, Stephanie Lavau, Nick Bingham and Simon Carter 2012

76 Reference to Morse Stephen S. 1993 in original.

77 Hinchliffe, Steve, John Allen, Stephanie Lavau, Nick Bingham and Simon Carter 2012, with reference to Morse, Stephen S, 1993

78 Hinchliffe, Steve, John Allen, Stephanie Lavau, Nick Bingham and Simon Carter 2012: 6 – 7, *italics added.*

79 Wolf, Meike 2012:117

necessarily *a priori* have been loaded with "mere life" to which "more life", that is pathogens, is added on the way through "impure" villages.

However, this does not happen. The Turkish National Strategy and the Global Strategy avoid enacting commercial or economic activity as a cause of HPAI avian influenza. This is ensured by various textual twists. By studying the strategies, I have so far seen how, by enacting avian influenza as an economic issue, spread goes *into* commercial sector as well as along commercial connections. In this way, avian influenza as an economic issue goes well together with avian influenza as an emerging disease issue studied above; both issues and their heterogeneous versions, as they are enacted in the strategy documents, are about spread, not origin. My analysis has shown that the economy is a victim that has to be protected. When the economy or commercial activities is about to become a cause, textual twists are, in the body text, efficiently restricting this to the informal sector. Rather than saying anything about how the commercial sector should be controlled in order to prevent the originating of HPAI, avian influenza control is becoming a matter of securing formal poultry trade; the strategies textualize *one* reality: namely that the commercial sector is a victim, and has the self-evident right to continue.

The stated "*Visions and Goals*" of the Global Strategy are in fact to "enhance a robust regional and international trade in poultry and poultry products".[80] For Vietnam, the strategy aims to "[set] up disease-free compartments from which unrestricted, safe trade in poultry products could be achieved".[81] Further on, "[t]his approach will enable Thailand to establish disease free compartments and to re-establish its lucrative export market (the world's fourth largest) within 1–3 years time."[82] For China and Indonesia, the aim is to "establish disease free compartments to trade safely in poultry products".[83] In order to reach its goals, the Turkish National Strategy stresses, in accordance with the Global Strategy, the "need ( … ) to enforce animal disease control measures in compliance with WTO/OIE and EU standards and thus to support the national trade and export of poultry and poultry products."[84]

---

80 FAO, OIE and WHO Nov: vii, 5, also in FAO, OIE and WHO 2005 May

81 FAO, OIE and WHO 2005 May: 7; 2005 Nov: 8

82 FAO, OIE and WHO 2005 May: 8; 2005 Nov: 9

83 *Op. cit.*

84 Ivanov, Yanko 2007: 72. This is in accordance with the Global Strategy which argues that the "application of OIE standards" is the solution: "The application of OIE standards relating to the international trade of poultry and poultry products will ( … ) assist in preventing the spread of HPAI virus across continents." (FAO, OIE and WHO 2005: May: iv; 2005 Nov: ix). Appendix 8 makes reference to the OIE/FAO's International Scientific Conference on Avian Influenza, OIE Paris, France, 7–8 April 2005 which highlights the importance of, and

An ambition of this book is to contribute to a re-ordering; so far, I have attempted to do this by drawing attention to some of the facts which remained in the appendix; facts that are of no concern in the body text. These facts are making emergence a matter of origin; moreover, as Hinchliffe et al. argue, these facts "emphasise the intra-actions that make disease a possibility in the first place."[85] Information in the Global Strategy's appendices suggest that such *intra-actions* are, in the case of HAPI, primarily take place in and among domestic poultry raised within intensive production systems. Furthermore, moving beyond the strategy documents, highly pathogenic avian influenza is commonly referred to as a *poultry disease*.[86] This calls attention to poultry and leads to the following question: how is avian influenza being enacted as a poultry issue in the strategies?

## A poultry issue – but no "poultry disease"

A piece of text taken from one of the strategy documents, a relevant excerpt, from which I could spin out my arguments, and which would connect my readers to these strategy documents, would fit well right here. It is in fact needed in order to attain a consistent structure for this chapter. Despite searching through the Global Strategy, I have yet to find the phrase "poultry disease" (or "disease in poultry" or "disease of poultry").[87] This "lack" of search result is no less of

faith in, standards and regulations for securing trade: "Preventing the spread of pathogens through international trade in animals and animal products is one of the primary missions of the World Organisation for Animal Health (OIE). This is accomplished by establishing and updating international standards and guidelines that prevent spread of pathogens while avoiding unjustified sanitary barriers." In addition, the appendix states, "The OIE works in close association with FAO in helping countries implement such standards and guidelines." The standards developed by the OIE are recognised as international standards for animal health and zoonoses by the Agreement on the Application of Sanitary and Phytosanitary Measures (SPS) of the World Trade Organization (WTO) and serves as a partner with the FAO/WHO Codex Alimentarius on animal production food safety. Implementation of these standards by Member Countries also has benefits for public health (including food safety) and improvement of animal production. In revised 2007 Global Strategy this is even more apparent. "Trade" is mentioned in the text when expressing the need to ensure "safe international trade in animals and animal products".

85 Hinchliffe, Steve et al. 2012: 7

86 Referring to HPAI as a "poultry disease" is common also in scientific publications published by OIE. There See e.g. Swayne, D. E. and D. L. Suarez 2000

87 The phrase "poultry diseases" is mentioned twice in the Turkish National Strategy; on one occasion it is mentioned in relation to legislation, whereby the laws regulating "poultry diseases" are explained: "[t]here are 3 notifiable poultry diseases in Turkey: AI, Newcastle disease and Salmonella (gallinarum & pullorum)." (Ivanov, Yanko 2007: 23)

an interesting result. Neither does it mean that the strategy documents are not enacting avian influenza as a poultry issue. On the contrary, "poultry" appears frequently in both the Global and the National Strategy. This section aims to analyse how avian influenza is enacted as a poultry issue in the strategy documents, if not as a poultry disease.

## Schematically ordering poultry as risky or secure

Table 3 in the back matter of the Global Strategy is literally *ordering* poultry according to five production systems. The table (inserted below) is explicitly referred to on three occasions in the body text, however, the five poultry production systems appear frequently throughout the Global Strategy and the Turkish National Strategy, with or without references to the table. The main parameters of the table are levels of "Biosecurity" and "Market outputs". The poultry production system categorized as "Industrial and integrated production" is characterized by a high-level of biosecurity, and, on the other end of this scale, "Village or backyard [p]roduction" is characterized by a low-level of biosecurity.[88] In this way, the table contributes to enacting poultry as perilous or safe according to which production practices they are part of.

The table itself is not passed on to the Turkish National Strategy, but it is still at work there. This is especially evident in the text that has been copied directly from the Global Strategy. Even though the table is missing in the National Strategy, the text is referring to it as if it were there, and thus carries on the same correlation between production system and biosecurity level.[89]

However, the Turkish National Strategy also makes use of a related definition of four poultry production sectors. This definition was put into practice 2004, the year before the table was first published, and was originally referring to poultry production systems in Asia.[90] The table on the other hand, can be traced back to a FAO report where a nearly identical table can be found.[91] According to the latter FAO report, the table was based on empirical studies from and used for analytical purposes in the study of the Asian countries, Cambodia,

88 FAO, OIE and WHO 2005 May: 26; 2005Nov: 33

89 The Turkish National Strategy explicitly refers to this table (Table 3) on two occasions (pp 32; 75), however, Table 3 in this document shows systems for manure disposal. While the poultry production system table did not make it to the Turkish National Strategy, the text refers to it and conveys the same correlation between system and biosecurity level.

90 FAO 2004 Sept.

91 Dolberg, Frands, Emmanuelle Guerne Bleich and Anni McLeod 2005. The table were based on and used for analytical purposes in the study of the Asian countries: Cambodia, Indonesia, Lao PDR and Vietnam.

**TABLE 3 - CHARACTERISTICS OF FOUR DIFFERENT POULTRY PRODUCTION SYSTEMS**

| **Characteristics** | **Poultry Production Systems** | | | | |
|---|---|---|---|---|---|
| **Parameter** | **Industrial and Integrated Production** | **Commercial poultry production** | | **Village or backyard Production** | |
| | | **Large Scale** | **Small-Scale** | **Poultry** | **Domestic ducks** |
| Production System | **System 1** | **System 2** | **System 3** | **System 4** | **System 5** |
| Biosecurity | High | Medium | Low | Low | Low |
| Market outputs | Export and urban | Urban/rural | Live urban/rural | Rural | Rural/Urban |
| Dependence on market for inputs | High | High | High | Medium | High |
| Dependence on market access | High | High | High | Medium | Medium |
| Location | Near capital and major cities | Near capital and major cities | Smaller towns and rural areas | Outdoors | Outdoors |
| Type of confinement | Indoors | Indoors | Indoors/Part-time outdoors | Not confined | Not confined |
| Housing | Closed | Closed | Closed/Open | Minimal | None |
| Contact with other poultry | None | None | Yes | | |
| Contact with domestic ducks | None | None | Yes | Yes | Yes |
| Contact with other domestic birds | None | None | Yes | Yes | Yes |
| Contact with wildlife | None | None | Yes | Yes | Yes |
| Veterinary services | Own Veterinarian | Pays for veterinary service | Pays for veterinary service | Irregular | Irregular |
| Source of medicine and vaccine | Market | Market | Market | Government, Market | Government, Market |
| Source of technical information | Company and associates | Sellers of inputs | Sellers of inputs | Govt. extension service | Govt. extension service |
| Source of financing | Banks and own | Banks and own | Banks and private | Private, occasionally Banks | Private, rarely Banks |
| Breed of poultry | Commercial | Commercial | Commercial/ Indigenous | Indigenous | Native |
| Food security of owner | High | High | High | Variable | High |

*Characteristics of poultry systems given in the Global Strtegy. (FAO, OIE and WHO 2005 May:26; 2005 Nov: 33)*

Indonesia, Lao PDR and Vietnam. The difference between the first version of the table and the one at work in the Global Strategy is that what is categorised as "Village and backyard production", which was originally System 4, has been divided into two categories: "Poultry" (System 4) and "Domestic ducks" (System 5). This may also explain why the table has five systems while the definition is still operating with four sectors.[92] Why do ducks receive a distinct role in the Global Strategy? I will shortly study this further. First, I would like to make a few more comments on how the table and the definitions contribute in ordering avian influenza as a poultry issue.

The table operates with 17 parameters characterizing the five different poultry production systems; hence, it specifies the three general parameters at work in the definitions: production system, biosecurity and market system. The largest industrial and integrated production system is characterized by "Closed", "Housing", and "None"; these are referenced with regards to the parameters that involve contact with other poultry, wild birds or wildlife. The opposite characteristic is given for the small production systems. Interestingly, the parameters characterizing market contact in both directions (inputs, output and access (i.e. roads)) do not have the same association with biosecurity. In this way, and I will argue this is very important, the table is enacting secure and insecure poultry production systems as a matter of housing and contact with other birds or wildlife – but not as a matter of market chains.

The table and the definition operate with the same direct relation between size and biosecurity level, but the way they give space for specificities, and the way specificities are working in the two, differs. The 17 subcategories at work in the table, coincide with, and thereby strengthen, the impression that market output and biosecurity levels are correlated; high output equals housing equals high level of biosecurity – and vice versa. By incorporating additional factors, and in this way being more specific, the table is strengthening certain correlations.

The definition, on the other hand, is less specific when it comes to parameters, as it operates with only three. Nonetheless, the definition allows slightly more text, and in this way it adds nuance to the specificities:

> The probability of infection is higher in production sectors 3 and 4 [small scale] than in sectors 1 and 2 [large scale]. However, if the virus does enter farms in sectors 1 and 2, infection may have a greater impact due to the concentration of susceptible poultry in these farms.

[92] The title of the table remains as "Characteristic of four…"; it is unclear whether the authors forgot to change it or if it was a conscious choice to keep the title to ensure harmony with the definition.

It is evident that the definition considers "impact" to be proportional to farm size; when the Turkish National Strategy brings along this definition, it provides space for this relation between impact and farm size in regards to biosecurity. *Emergence*, in the sense of *origin,* of HPAI virus strains could have been a concern here. However, as we have already seen, the strategies are about something that already exists; hence, the "impact" at stake is *spread.*[93] The quoted text above is followed by this solution: "It is possible to reduce the risk of an HPAI outbreak and to improve control over a disease situation by changing *industry practices* (e.g. poultry production, transportation and marketing) that facilitate viral spread."[94] While changing "industry practises" is considered the solution for sector 1 and 2 farms, sector 3 and 4 represents "[c]onstraints to implementing biosecurity measures":

> In Turkey, a significant percentage of farmers keep poultry in village/backyard production systems, characterised by local indigenous breeds adapted to scavenging habits. Measures to increase biosecurity are difficult to put in place ( ... ) Providing fencing or coops to keep backyard poultry enclosed in some areas could be an initial stage in which to implement biosecurity. However, being on the onus of the owner to find or purchase feed for the poultry will require intensive and well adapted communication campaigns.[95]

What we see here is that physical barriers between domestic and wild are pivotal; large industrial productions systems are regarded as possible to control, *contrary* to small backyard flocks, which are considered as *almost* ungovernable. Consequently, the concept of *biosecurity* contributes to enacting all aspects of poultry and their way of living as good or bad, safe or risky, secure or insecure. Operating with the table and the definitions, the Global Strategy and the Turkish National Strategy reproduce the same relation between size and biosecurity.

In the table, "poultry" is *including*; as a category it embraces all kinds of domesticated birds kept for economic or nutritious utility purposes. "Domestic ducks" are standing out as the only type of poultry that are specified in the table. What is it about ducks, in the Global Strategy, that makes them so

93 A parallel can be drawn to Harris and Keil's (2007) argument about neoliberalism moving the focus from prevention to treatment.

94 Ivanov, Yanko 2007: 55–56, *italics added.*

95 Ivanov, Yanko 2007: 62–63. Interestingly the hesitant backyard poultry keepers that appear in the Turkish National Strategy, who are in need of "intensive and well adapted communication campaigns" gain support in a FAO document published one year later, titled *Biosecurity for Highly Pathogenic Avian Influenz*. Here it is emphasized that previous advice must be fundamentally "reassessed". (FAO 2008: 22–23). Geerlings (2006) also raises these issues in her assessment of HPAI socio-economic impacts in Turkey.

special that they deserve their own column appointing sector characteristics exclusively for them?

## Asian ducks: Virus carriers, silent hosts, source of infection and legitimizers for a global strategy

The part of the Global Strategy that is presenting*Infected Countries in South, East and Southeast Asia* is a good place to get an impression of the role of ducks in relation to avian influenza in this region.[96] The presence of ducks in this section is striking; ducks are the only poultry that are specified. In this section, reviewing the outbreaks that had already occurred when the Draft version was published (that was prior to the spread beyond Asia), I was not able to detect any other avian species such as "chicken", "turkeys", "geese" or "quail". Neither does the term "wild birds" occur here. Ducks, on the other hand, appear frequently.

Thailand and China for example, both have a "vast duck population".[97] Furthermore, the Global Strategy states, "Indonesia also harbours a large duck population"; similarly, Vietnam's "large carrier duck populations" appears significant in the description of the avian influenza situation. In China, ducks "[act] as a source of infection for terrestrial poultry".[98] In Thailand they are "acting as a host reservoir for the virus, [which] needs to be urgently addressed",[99] and "carrier duck reservoirs remain a constant threat to re-infection."[100] Also, ducks in Vietnam "act as huge reservoir for infection."[101] In this way, ducks possess the role as the "source of infection", "reservoir" and "threat to re-infection".

Moving to Appendix 2, which provides technical information on the HPAI virus in Asia, "the large (660 million) domestic duck population in PR China" is a cause for concern.[102] While previous experience with HPAI has shown that these viruses cause "serious mortality", this was not the case this time.[103] Rather, this time "[t]he virus ( . . . ) spread rapidly" among the ducks, but, contrary to previous experience, it was "causing little or no disease symptoms."[104]

[96] FAO, OIE and WHO 2005 May: 7; 2005 Nov: 7
[97] FAO, OIE and WHO 2005 May: iv; 2005 Nov: viii
[98] FAO, OIE and WHO 2005 May: 8; 2005 Nov: 9
[99] FAO, OIE and WHO 2005 May: iv; 2005 Nov: viii
[100] FAO, OIE and WHO 2005 May: 8; 2005 Nov: 9
[101] FAO, OIE and WHO 2005 May: 7; 2005 Nov: 8
[102] FAO, OIE and WHO 2005 May: 37; 2005 Nov: 47
[103] FAO, OIE and WHO 2005 May: 37; 2005 Nov: 47
[104] FAO, OIE and WHO 2005 May: 37; 2005 Nov: 47

This makes ducks silent hosts, or "an important H5N1 reservoir"[105] and "a source of infection".[106] As pointed out, also in the body text of the Global Strategy, "[a]ffected domestic ducks show lower morbidity and mortality than chickens but become virus shedders. Recent studies in Viet Nam indicate that close to 20% of asymptomatic domestic ducks in the Mekong Delta shed significant quantities of HPAI virus."[107] Furthermore,

> [T]he widespread circulation of the H5N1 in domestic ducks and terrestrial poultry has resulted into the selection of more aggressive Z genotype with a Z+ strain infective to humans and spreading to Thailand, Viet Nam and more recently to Cambodia. While this is a clear and present threat to global poultry industry and public health, the constant and rapid evolution of the virus necessitates a global approach to controlling the disease.[108]

Here we see that the bodies of "ducks and terrestrial poultry" enact places where H5N1 virus may reside, develop and turn "more aggressive". This is not a problem confined to the bodies of the birds; it also affects their surroundings: Epidemiological investigations "estimated that infected waterfowl were excreting virus for as long as 17 days following infection, causing a huge contamination of the environment."[109] However, this latter epidemiological finding remained in the appendix; it is not presented as a matter of concern in the body text, thus HPAI does not become an environmental- or a pollution issue. Nonetheless, the ducks in the Global Strategy are enacted as "a clear and present threat to global poultry industry and public health". As we see in the latter excerpt, the "evolution of the virus", in which this strategy makes it clear that ducks play an important and special role, also "necessitates a global approach". In this way, ducks play a critical role in justifying a global strategy.

All the places in the Draft version where ducks have been reported to be present remain unchanged in the Final version. In the text, which has been added to the Final version, ducks hardly appear.[110] Ducks have been important actors in Asia, but how is their role affected when the virus enters Europe? Moving to the National Strategy, in what ways do ducks contribute to enacting avian influenza as a poultry issue in the Turkish setting?

---

105 FAO, OIE and WHO 2005 May: 12; 2005 Nov: 16

106 FAO, OIE and WHO 2005 May: 8; 2005 Nov: 9

107 FAO, OIE and WHO 2005 May: 18; 2005 Nov: 24

108 FAO, OIE and WHO 2005 May: 3; 2005 Nov: 3

109 FAO, OIE and WHO 2005 May: 37; 2005 Nov: 47

110 In the added text, "ducks" are mentioned 4 times (in contrast to "wild birds" which are mentioned 32 times).

## Moving to Turkey: Ducks remain ducks or turn into poultry

"As long as facts are apples and oranges, one cannot generalize across them", Anna Tsing writes; "one must first see them as 'fruits' to make general claims."[111] This is one way of making the Asian ducks of the Global Strategy mobile and able to be move, and to act in the National Strategy. This is about generalisation; the Asian ducks are not turning into fruit when they enter the Turkish National Strategy, but into "poultry"; a general term that also covers other domestic birds primarily used for consumption, such as chickens or hens. The latter are particularly relevant to Turkey. Domestic ducks play a very limited role in Turkey compared to how their role in Asian countries is enacted in the Global Strategy.[112] When "ducks", in the Global Strategy, turn into "poultry" in the Turkish National Strategy, this involves a transfer of the critical qualities associated with ducks, *via poultry,* onto chickens and hens. This is happening because reading "poultry" in a Turkish setting will primarily be associated with chicken and hens, *piliç* and *tavuk* – the main kind of poultry in Turkey.

One way of making ducks able to move across strategies is thus to allow the general (here "poultry" or "backyard poultry farming") to raise above the particular (ducks).[113] When Asian *ducks* turn into*poultry* in the Turkish National Strategy, they bring along some specificities and qualities while others are no more made to matter.[114] What they bring along is the free range nature of the production system to which they belong. *Free range ducks* are turning into *free range poult*ry or *backyard poultry*, which, in Turkish, is *köy tavuk*, which literally means *village chicken*. Furthermore, they bring along their *general* role as a challenge to disease control and eradication. Specificities related to farming systems, for example flock size or density, and physiological qualities are details that are lost on the way from the Global Strategy to the Turkish National Strategy; the physiological specificities of the particular virus-duck relations are applied to a general virus-poultry relation.

---

111 Tsing, Anna 2005: 89

112 According to official national statistics from 2005, 925.900 ton of broiler meat was produced (slaughtered) and only two tonnes of duck meat (http://www.turkstat.gov.tr/VeriBilgi.do?tb_id=46&ust_id=13, *read* 25.11.2011). As highlighted in the Turkish National Strategy (Ivanov, Yanko 2007) backyard poultry are not registered, however, my general impression during field trips across Turkey is that what is commonly referred to as backyard poultry, *köy tavuğu* which literally means village hen or chicken, is primarily chicken. The few studies that I have found regarding backyard poultry in Turkey also support my impressions (Please see Durutan, Nedret and Okan Cüneyt n.d; 2006; Geerlings, Ellen 2006)

113 Tsing, Anna 2005: 89. See e.g. Ivanov, Yanko 2007: 40

114 Regarding "specificities" see Law, John 2004

As illustrated above, the strategies recognise these specificities as being crucial in regard to emergence and spread. Nevertheless, they did not move well from the appendix to the body text of the Global Strategy. As ducks are turning into backyard poultry as they (re)appear in the National Strategy, backyard poultry hold, including the hens involved in this practice, are also turning more risky; through generalisation risk factors are accumulating and all the "apples and oranges", chickens *as* ducks, are becoming *as risky as the sum* of poultry.

Ducks are not always turning into poultry as they move across strategies. At several places in the document text ducks remain ducks in the Turkish National strategy.[115] Sometimes the relation to place is explicitly mentioned and maintained in a way that allow the ducks to remain Asian when they reappear in the Turkish National Strategy: "Twenty percent of clinically normal ducks in the Mekong Delta of Viet Nam were found harbouring the HPAI virus".[116] In other incidents, they enter the Turkish National Strategy without any spatial connection: "The fact that domestic ducks can act as a "silent" reservoir has removed the warning signal of a risk".[117] Domestic ducks are enacted as "silent hosts" several places in the Global Strategy. The exact sentence presented here does not appear in the Global Strategy; rather it can be traced back to the WHO publication titled, *Responding to the Avian Influenza Pandemic Threat*, which is also based on experiences from Asia.[118] With this sentence, ducks are carrying on the general role as "a 'silent host'". I will argue that these ducks are what Latour addresses as i*mmutable mobiles*; they keep their shape and they work in the same way when they move from one place to another.

On other occasions, we find, what Law and Mol refer to as "displacements which depend on mutability instead of, or as well as, immutability."[119] These are the ducks that smoothly *adapt* to Turkish conditions by small, but efficient textual adjustments; this is indicated by text I have set in *italics*:

**The Global Strategy writes:**
The nature of *farming systems in some countries, where domestic ducks are moved in flocks over long distances from province to province to feed on harvested rice fields,* plays *a major* role in the transmission and maintenance of the HPAI virus, and in compromising the traditional control measures of active surveillance'culling of infected

[115] "Duck" appears 38 times the Turksih National Strategy (Ivanov, Yanko 2007).

[116] Ivanov, Yanko 2007: 40; Also added in the Final version of the Global Strategy (FAO, OIE, WHO 2005 Nov: 17)

[117] Ivanov, Yanko 2007: 76

[118] WHO 2005: 5

[119] Law, John and Annemarie Mol 2001: 619

flocks and imposition of biosecurity. (...)Preventing the intermingling of ducks and domestic poultry would serve to significantly reduce HPAI transmission.[120]

**The Turkish National Strategy re-writes:**
The nature of*backyard poultry farming in Turkey, where free-grazing ducks share the same habitats with the wild birds during the day and come back home at night mingling with the other domestic poultry, could* play *an important* role in the transmission and maintenance of the HPAI virus, and in compromising the traditional control measures of active surveillance, culling of infected flocks and imposition of biosecurity. *Therefore* preventing the intermingling of ducks and domestic poultry would serve to significantly reduce the risk of HPAI transmission.[121]

In the first text taken from the Global Strategy, Asian ducks contribute to spread due to a particular farming practice "*where domestic ducks are moved in flocks over long distances*".[122] In the second excerpt taken from the Turkish National Strategy, Asian ducks are turned into Turkish ducks and made to cohabit with "wild birds" and "other domestic poultry", with the latter not being further specified. In this way, ducks no longer play a dominant role, as they did in the Global Strategy.

Adjusted to Turkish conditions, ducks have become few, and they are living among various poultry species; when the text moves from the Global Strategy to the Turkish National Strategy, the practices and physical location of "ducks" alter; It is no longer a *large flock moving from province to province*, but *small groups of ducks taken out in the morning to grass, most likely by a nearby pond or a creek, and then home again in the evening.*[123] Again, according to Law and Mol, this is a kind of "globalization [that] is not about networks but about fluidities. About movements that go more easily if there is less control. About

[120] FAO, OIE, WHO Nov 2005: 16–17; with the exception of the last sentence: May 2005: 12.

[121] Ivanov, Yanko 2007: 40

[122] Ian Scoones and Paul Forster (2008) also mention the special role or the "particular challenges in some parts of Asia" related to "free grazing ducks in rice cropping areas". Importantly, Scoones and Forster emphasize that "these situations are often highly particular, and dependent on a wide range of factors from local ecological ones (...) the structure of the industry (...) the economics of production (...) and the regulatory and policy environment"(2008:17). When textualized, "ducks" move from Asia to Turkey via the Global Strategy, they are enacted as "particular agents of spread". Significantly, Scoons and Forster point at how "[t]he focus on 'risk groups' (...) may remove the emphasis from the wider context the epidemic's 'configuration' in Rosenberg's terms." (2008:37 with reference to Rosenberg Charles. E. 1992)

[123] In addition to personal observations made during my field trips (as presented in Chapter 2), Durutan, Nedret and Cüneyt Okan 2006 and Geerlings, Ellen 2006 provide valuable accounts of backyard poultry in Turkey.

things that take on the shape of their surroundings. That are adaptable."[124] Moreover, what I have shown here is just how the rather marginally present ducks in Turkey have contributed to adapting text to the Turkish setting; while the large flocks of Asian ducks in the first text are associated with the potential regional spread of the virus, the small groups of Turkish ducks in the second text are given the role as potential bridges between wild and domestic poultry locally. These are the details, the *specificities*, that are adjustable and adjusted, in ways that make "ducks" *mutable mobiles*;[125] flock size and movement patterns, factors commonly considered crucial to virology and epidemiology, change as "ducks" move from Asia to Turkey via the Global Strategy. Again to paraphrase Law and Mol, "ducks" are adaptable and adapted; they are *fluid* and "*take the shape of their surroundings*".

However, this analysis also shows how ducks contribute in *shaping their surroundings*. While the Asian ducks are turned into Turkish ducks in the first part of this second excerpt, the rest of the text can remain nearly unchanged. In this way, the "ducks" maintain their central "role in the transmission and maintenance of the HPAI virus (. . . )". Hence, "ducks" are also immutable mobiles; the version of "ducks" as being critical in relation to HPAI keeps its shape as it moves from Asia to Turkey; they are immutable mobiles in that their epidemiological role remains the same as they are re-textualized and contribute to making the Turkish HPAI reality.

Fundamental to both the Global Strategy and the Turkish National Strategy is the idea of controllability.[126] Approaching avian influenza as a poultry issue and studying the schematically defined version of this, I have traced the relation between production system, or sector, and biosecurity level: closed farming systems are enacted as safe or biosecure and possible to control, while open systems are enacted as bio*in*secure and harder to control. As text moves from the Global Strategy to the Turkish National Strategy, control becomes less about physiological features, flock size or specific farming systems in which they are part of, but simply about domestic wild interference. Ducks are not mobile because of their particular physiology which in the Global Strategy made them "silent hosts" and virus "reservoirs"; they are so because they are

---

[124] Law, John and Annemarie Mol 2001: 619

[125] As above, Law's (2004a) advice and convincing argument illustrate why we should pay attention to the specificities mentioned here.

[126] For the case of readability and simplicity, I refer to these documents as the Turkish National Strategy and the Global Strategy, but it is worthwhile to remember their full titles (where "control" is a central concept in both): *Strategy for Highly Pathogenic Avian Influenza Preparedness and Control in Turkey* and*A Global Strategy for the Progressive Control of Highly Pathogenic Avian Influenza (HPAI)*

*free range poultry*. In Asia, according to the Global Strategy, "domestic ducks" are free range in the sense that they are kept on open rice fields. In Turkey, as enacted in the Turkish National Strategy, the avian influenza problem is about "backyard poultry farming" where "free-grazing ducks" *may* co-exist together with "other domestic poultry". As mentioned in the opening of this chapter, the Global Strategy encourages individual countries to "have a complete plan of action and ( . . . ) to implement it under the particular conditions in the country."[127] Studying avian influenza as a poultry issue has made two things clear: the measures to address the disease have been fitted to the Turkish setting, and the core of the problem, which in Asia was closely associated with ducks, has, in the Turkish context, been turned into a chicken or hen problem.

## A human health issue

Veterinary and Public health services should work together to improve national, regional and global health security. Public health services should support the agriculture sector/veterinary services in order to control and eliminate the disease at source and to protect farmers and workers from animal infection in the most efficient and efficacious manner.[128]

The interesting thing happening in this text, which is taken from the Global Strategy, is not only that HPAI is necessitating collaboration between veterinary and public health services. It is also establishing a vertical relationship between these sectors where "[p]ublic health services should support the agriculture sector/veterinary services", rather than the reverse. This challenges the common, hierarchical notion that humans are above animals; thus it encourages reflections on how human-animal relations are enacted within the intersectoral framework of *One World, One Health*, given these strategy documents are a part of this initiative.[129] In order to analyse how avian influenza is enacted

[127] Ivanov, Yanko 2007: pp 6–7. The first part of this excerpt can also be found in the Global Strategies (FAO, OIE and WHO 2005 May: ii; 2005 Nov: vi). As it has been slightly rewritten to make it suitable for the Turkish National Strategy, "this document" has been changed to "the global strategy"

[128] FAO, OIE and WHO 2005 May: 51; 2005 Nov: 63

[129] For accounts of human-animal relations, and more specifically on how the "hierarchy where animals served human purposes for achieving higher ends" is enacted through the Norwegian penal code, see Asdal, Kristin 2008c; on the changing nature of human-animal relations, see Asdal, Kristin 2012. In relation to avian influenza, Natalie Porters' study on avian influenza in Viet Nam shows how the hierarchical ordering of humananimal relations also is at work in the relationship between medical practitioners. Her study highlights a number of conflicts that arose when veterinaries and public health workers were supposed to cooperate,

as a human health issue, I will examine three specific relations in which avian influenza is performing within the strategy documents. First, I will study the human health issue as a matter of pandemic; I will explore how humans operate within the strategies, both as individuals and as a population. The second relation is that between non-humans and humans as avian influenza is becoming a matter of zoonosis. Finally, I trace how the human health issue is becoming, and how it is working as, a matter of product-consumer relation.

## The risk of pandemic: How numbers are making avian influenza matter and instigate the development of strategies

> With the present situation, the potential of the HPAI virus to become transmissible among humans is of serious concern to the global community. If the virus adapts itself to human-to human transmission, millions of lives may be threatened. The WHO estimates that millions of people could die of HPAI, should a human pandemic occur. Considering the potential for this scenario, [it is] recommended that a global strategy be developed and implemented to help stem the broad negative impact of the disease.[130]

In this section of the Global Strategy, HPAI is considered as a human health issue of "serious concern to the global community" in that the virus may potentially lead to a human pandemic where "millions of people could die". The numbers contribute to materialise and stabilize avian influenza as an economic issue, and in this way legitimizes the need for a strategy; numbers or "estimates" are also effective in establishing avian influenza as a major human health concern requiring, as the text above says, *a global strategy*. As above, global public health concerns accompany economic concerns when answering the following rhetorical question: "Why a global strategy?[131]

> The continuing outbreaks of highly pathogenic avian influenza (HPAI) ( … ) have raised serious global public health concerns. Over ( … ) a hundred people have contracted the infection, of which close to 60 have died since May 2005.[132]

---

but where the latter lacked respect for the veterinarians' professional capacity claiming that they were "failed medical students" (Porter 2013a: 136). Through the concept of *biopower*, Porter also explores the role of veterinaries in defining public health policy, and how they interfere in how people should conduct in their poultry-rearing practices. While the role of veterinarians is institutionally strengthened, Porter shows, with reference to Foucault, how their authority is undermined through acts of "resistance and counter-conduct" (Porter, Natalie 2014 *forthcoming*)

[130] FAO, OIE, WHO 2005 May: iii FAO, OIE AND WHO 2005 Nov: vii

[131] FAO, OIE, WHO 2005 Nov.: vii

[132] *Op. cit.*

These numbers, or more precisely – by being turned into numbers – these "people", who have "contracted" or even "died" from "the [HPAI] infection", serve to justify the Global Strategy. By being enacted as a group, these people are *not* individuals bringing in specific experiences for the strategy to draw upon; it is not their individually lived lives and concerns that matter.[133] Unlike poultry or ducks, humans do not play multiple roles in the strategies; as previously mentioned, poultry and ducks are enacted, for example, as reservoirs, sources of infection, silent hosts and so on. One implication following from this is: by *not* paying attention to the individual experiences of the people who have contracted or died from HPAI infection and the numbers through which they are enacted, the strategies fail to make even the most obvious matters related to the human pandemic, for example, access to and the quality of public health services, a matter of concern. In contrast, "*Inadequate veterinary services – a major weakness*" is a matter of concern that receives its own section in the Global Strategy under just this heading.[134]

There are several contributing factors that make this relatively small, though no less unfortunate, group of HPAI victims unique. One major concern, in the strategies and elsewhere, is that these people – these humans – have apparently contracted the virus directly from poultry, and – most significantly – each new human infection represents a new opportunity for the avian influenza virus to re-assort or mutate and become enabled to move directly between people. If, in this process, the virus would also maintain its lethal capacity, the pandemic would be a real risk. This leads me to the second relation in which avian influenza is enacted as a human health issue; what is commonly referred to as the zoonotic nature of the virus, is making bodily relations between avian and human species a matter of concern that demands careful consideration.

## The zoonotic nature: Connecting institutional bodies

> Given the zoonotic and transboundary nature of the disease, appropriate linkages and policies need to be established among a number of ministries and groups at the national (e.g., provincial, district, community and farmer levels), regional and international levels to enhance the coordination of HPAI control.[135]

The text quoted here appears in the Global Strategy and the Turkish National Strategy. The zoonotic (and transboundary) nature of HPAI in this text con-

133 Please refer to this discussion in the introduction of this volume. Among relevant references is Moser, Ingunn 2003; 2005; 2011.

134 FAO, OIE, WHO 2005 Nov.: 15

135 Global Strategy 2005 May: 13; 2005 Nov: 1; Ivanov, Yanko 2007: 64

tributes to materializing a need for intersectoral (and international) "linkages" and "coordination". When avian influenza is enacted as a zoonosis or as a zoonotic disease throughout both the Global Strategy and the Turkish National Strategy, it becomes an administrative and organizational matter, with only one exception: when the zoonotic nature of avian influenza is part of something "bigger", namely the whole group of (re)emerging zoonotic diseases. The term zoonosis commonly refers to pathogens such as viruses, bacteria, parasites or prions that are able to move (or be moved) from non-human animals to humans.[136] Rather than connecting avian and human bodies per se, this capacity does, in the strategies, contribute to linking or connecting institutional bodies in charge of governing human and non-human bodies. In other words, the inter-special concern of zoonosis in the strategies involves turning avian influenza into a matter of intersectoral cooperation.

Intersectoral cooperation is enacted as general, organizational and institutional arrangements, without further details about what these arrangements should involve or how they should work. In order to see how inter-special virus movement or zoonotic virus flow is enacted more specifically in these strategy documents, we have to leave the places where the term "zoonosis" or "zoonotic disease" is at work, and rather study the places where the more general term "human health" is at work.

It is in relation to "human health" that we can study how inter-special circulations are enacted in the strategies, and more specifically, how they are made to be governed and secured. Also, it is here that we can trace the vital twist: when the strategies are handling the issue of human health, humans are turned into consumers and avian species are enacted as poultry products. After studying how avian influenza as a human health issue is enacted as a pandemic and as zoonosis, I will round off my exploration of this heterogeneous issue by studying what avian influenza becomes when it is enacted as a matter of product-consumer relation.

### A human health issue: Securing consumers, products and markets

Both the Global Strategy and the Turkish National Strategy emphasise the right to safe poultry products. The Turkish National Strategy stresses the importance of "assurance to consumers that product is derived from disease free sources".[137] Similarly, the Draft version of the Global Strategy advocates "im-

136 WHO/FAO/OIE 2004: *Report of the WHO/FAO/OIE joint consultation on emerging zoonotic diseases*

137 Ivanov, Yanko 2007: 53

proved food safety for consumers", and the Final version explicitly adds that there is a need for "improved food safety and decreased health hazards".[138] According to both the Global Strategy and the Turkish National Strategy, the health of consumers should be protected from any potential harm caused by poultry products.

The Turkish National Strategy emphasises that consumers of poultry products should have "confidence".[139] This specifically refers to commercially marketed poultry meat. Much like in the case of poultry production above, communication is central in terms of consumption. This also receives special attention in the Turkish National Strategy. For example it emphasises that "epidemiological understanding of the determinants of HPAI transmission is essential for setting sound control strategies and to inform public communication to minimise disruption to the poultry industry and maintain *consumer confidence*."[140] Furthermore, one of the central goals expressed in the Turkish National Strategy is to "stabilise national poultry production and trade, rehabilitate exports of poultry and poultry products, [and to] increase consumer confidence in food safety."[141] In order to reach this goal, the Turkish National Strategy calls for "[m]assive communication campaigns":

> Massive communication campaigns are needed to sensitise communities to the risks to health and livelihoods and the means of minimising those risks. However, it is essential that these be conducted with sensitivity to the damage that inappropriate messages can cause to commercial poultry production. One component of public awareness campaigns should be to *educate the public on the risks of acquiring human infection by indicating that poultry can be consumed safely if the appropriate precautions are taken*.[142]

Here, the Turkish National Strategy emphasises that communication campaigns should convey *both the risk and product safety at the same time*. In this way, the Turkish National Strategy attempts to make protection of both human health and the market for commercial poultry production one, intertwined goal. This alliance between poultry consumption and commercial production contributes to producing *one* possible version of safe consumption; that is, the consumption of commercial poultry products. In this way, non-commercial poultry, commonly referred to as backyard poultry or *köy tavuğu* in Turkey, is

[138] FAO, OIE AND WHO 2005 May: 21; 2005 Nov: 26
[139] Ivanov, Yanko 2007: 8, 38
[140] Ivanov, Yanko 2007: 38, *italics added.*
[141] Ivanov, Yanko 2007: 8
[142] Ivanov, Yanko 2007: 64,*italics added.*

not included by the Turkish National Strategy as it attempts to create a version safe human-animal relationships for the purposes of consumption.

Studying avian influenza in the strategies as a matter of product-consumer relation has enabled me to trace how making poultry products safe is becoming a major concern. Moreover, safe poultry is not about healthy poultry in itself or animal welfare (the latter not being mentioned at all in the strategies); rather, the aim is to (re-)establish consumer confidence. However, consumer confidence, based on a healthy and satisfied public, is not a goal in itself either; both avian and human species, enacted as poultry products and consumers thereof, become subordinate to "commercial poultry production". By studying avian influenza as a human health issue, the "commercial poultry production" emerges as the primary actor that has to be *secured*. This resembles what we saw in the previous sections, that the economy and the commercial poultry sector are in need of protection against "market shocks".

## Drawing things together

This chapter has been developed through a great deal of re-reading, analysing, re-writing and editing. After a long process filled with struggles and (believe it or not) fun, the strategy documents and this chapter have been tamed, and empirical and analytical issues have emerged. These strategy documents were among the first empirical sites I explored at the beginning of the project, and my relation to them has changed with time. At first, these documents were, on the one hand, surprisingly easy to read: they possess clear language and an orderly structure, special concepts are kept to a minimum and they are not excessively long. On the other hand, they are impermeable: every word of these documents appears to be important, the texts appears balanced, uncontroversial and modest both when acknowledging insecurity and emphasising that updated versions would be necessary as new knowledge was expected to emerge. After extensive engagement with these documents, they have turned into complex sites of investigation; the documents have become sites that I continuously return to in order to study some of all the exciting things that are still (!) *happening* within and between them. Except for my markings and notes, the documents are still the same as those I downloaded at the very beginning of this project.[143] However, they are also different. We are different; the documents and I have changed; we are changing each other.

*How* this change has occurred is closely related to three analytical moves. At the beginning, I was looking for a description of *what* avian influenza is within these documents. Unsurprisingly, I could trace several *perspectives* on *what* avian influenza is, in these documents written by various actors responsible for animal health, human health trade and global and national interests. So what? What sense does it make to identify these different perspectives? After moving between the strategy documents and theoretical literature, mainly related to the field of STS, I realized that it would be interesting to analyse *how* these perspectives work together, and no less, *how* they are enacted in the first place; thus, I attended to the ordering and re-ordering of *issues* within and between these documents. In order to do this, I had to pay careful attention to the *processes* that take place in and between the texts; the processes that made and re-made the *issues* in the first place. And, please note the important twist happening when changing from perspectives to issues. A further explanation might be necessary, and so I will provide one, as I now also clarify the second and interrelated analytical move that made me get a grip on these documents; that has been to study the documents in parallel.

Juxtaposing the documents and then seeing the same words in different places, for example in the two versions of the Global Strategy and/or in the Turkish National Strategy, enabled me to trace how the same words work differently; namely, how the words, to paraphrase Asdal, are *textualizing different realities* at the different places they are put to work. So, my point is: these texts are not simply presenting various perspectives; the texts are *making issues*; they are *enacting a multiple reality*.[144]

The third analytical move has involved oscillating between the realities enacted in and by the Turkish National Strategy and "the reality out there", at various places in Turkey. What I witnessed and heard (people's voices as well as crowing roosters) during my fieldwork in Turkey, influenced what I saw in and how I could work with the documents. One of the clearest examples is how, subsequent to one of my field trips, I developed an interest in studying the impact of text as it moves from the Global Strategy which is heavily in-

[143] I had already read the Global Strategy when I wrote the project proposal. During my first field trip to Ankara, one of my informants was busy writing the Turkish National Strategy. I was eager to receive a copy of the document, which he promised to e-mail me, but at that time, I had no idea about how much time and mental energy this document required.

[144] I draw closely on the analytical arguments presented by Mol, Annemarie 2005 [1999] and developed further in Mol, Annemarie 2002.

fluenced by the experiences of avian influenza in Asia, to the Turkish strategy. More specifically, how could the "vast duck population" predominant in the textualization of Thailand and China, or the experiences from "Viet Nam and other countries with large duck populations" be fitted into the Turkish strategy? The outbreak places in particular, and the general pattern of poultry hold and production I had come to know from my field trips in Turkey and additional research, appeared quite different to the places enacted in the Global Strategy. In Turkey, ducks are marginal. Rather, there are hens; they are comprised of either a small flock of 6 to 60 free rangeing birds, or they are part of the commercial sector where several thousand hens are enclosed in a poultry house. Moving between the different strategy documents and my experiences in Turkey, I became aware of the contrasts between Asian and Turkish poultry hold; consequently, this influenced the manner in which I read and analysed the texts. As I have shown in this chapter, the Asian ducks have found their way into the Turkish National Strategy: they appear as Asian ducks or they simply turn into the more general category of "backyard poultry". Hence, they have contributed to enacting avian influenza as a poultry issue in various ways in the Turkish National Strategy.

Following *how* avian influenza is *becoming a matter of concern* in various ways is about studying the emergence of heterogeneous realities. In other words, by studying ordering of issues, I have also traced how issues are enacted in different versions and how these multiple issues and their heterogeneous versions work together – or not! – within the *relational space* offered by these documents.[145]

My analysis shows how that which concerns emergence, in the sense of origin, remain in the appendix, with the effect that the circumstances and processes in regards to how LPAI are turning highly pathogenic is not a matter of concern in the body text of these documents. In the body text, avian influenza *is* already highly pathogenic. While it is mentioned as matters of fact in the appendix how HPAI develops within large scale intensive farming systems, and that markets and trade are playing a role in origin *and* spread, this does not become matters of concern in the body text of the strategies. In this way, the economy is not enacted as a cause for, but a victim of, avian influenza; when avian influenza is enacted as an economic issue, it is the negative, even "devastating", consequences *on* the economy that is the concern – not the role of

[145] As mentioned in the introduction of this chapter, the concept of "'relational space" is borrowed from Asdal (2014); on regarding multiple issues and heterogeneous versions see Mol, Annemarie 2002.

commercial poultry production systems in emergence and spread.[146] The fact that the genetic processes that may turn low pathogenic viruses into a highly pathogenic ones is not a concern, together with the unquestioned concern related to re-establish "safe trade in poultry", contribute to enacting avian influenza as a poultry issue in a particular way.[147] Analyzing what I have called schematically ordered poultry, I have traced how a form is enacting poultry production systems as biosecure or bio*in*secure; the bioseure are large and characterized by closed/housing, while small scale production is enacted as bio*in*secure due to how this practice is associated with free ranging or outdoor farming and contact with the wild. In this way, through the schematic ordering of poultry production systems, large-scale production is enacted as secure while small-scale production is enacted as insecure. Drawing together the matters of economic concern and the biosecure poultry production system enacted through the form, the strategies are producing a reality where big is beautiful when it comes to poultry production systems and biosecurity.

Finally, when studying avian influenza as a human health issue, it becomes clear that the heterogeneous version through which avian influenza is enacted as a human health issue contributes to stabilize the same reality. My analysis shows how humans are enacted as consumers in these documents; in relation to human health, poultry products ought to be safe – neither for the meat quality itself, nor for the wellbeing of the poultry but, as the Turkish National Strategy emphasises, to ensure "consumer confidence".[148] Furthermore, when avian influenza is enacted as a human or public health issue, this contributes to legitimizing the strategy, either as a pandemic threat where numbers make the issue big and real, or as a zoonosis which calls for intersectoral cooperation.

By studying how these four heterogeneous issues are enacted and how they co-exist within the relational space of these strategy documents, I have traced how the avian influenza reality has been ordered through this intersectoral cooperation. Initially, I raised the question: what does avian influenza become when organizations in charge of human health (WHO), food and agriculture (FAO) and animal health (OIE) agree upon a common understanding of a

146 "Devastating" is used in the Global Strategy at two occasion in relations to economy FAO, OIE and WHO 2005 May: 4, Appendix 1; FAO, OIE and WHO 2005 Nov: 4, Appendix 1.

147 FAO, OIE and WHO 2005 May: 21, 30 (Table 6); 2005 Nov: 27, 40 (Table6). In regards to Thailand in particular, a stated goal is "to re-establish its lucrative export market (the world's fourth largest) within 1–3 years time." (FAO, OIE and WHO 2005 May: 8; 2005 Nov: 9.

148 Ivanov, Yanko 2007: 8, 38. Low consumer confidence is also mentioned in Appendix 3of the Global Strategy in relation to economic impacts in Asian countries/Viet Nam. (FAO, OIE and WHO 2005 May; 2005 Nov)

global problem, something that must (?) be a precondition for formulating a common strategy? Throughout my analysis I have shown how the strategies are enacting avian influenza as complex concern.[149] Nonetheless, the three organisations as well as the Turkish national authorities, manage to enact a single goal through these strategy documents. Based on careful analysis, I will argue that it is just the complexity that enables "drawing things together", with the words of Latour.[150]

As my detailed analyses has shown, the different issues, and versions thereof, work well together; these documents are strategies *against* avian influenza, but at the same time strategies *for* biosecure poultry production; the documents also clearly specify how biosecure poultry production ought to be managed – that is closed and on a large scale – as well as how it ought not to be managed – that is free range and on a small scale. Making the issue of origin, both for HPAI as well as other zoonotic and/or transboundary animal diseases, a matter of concern, the strategies could have advocated alternative sources of protein. As this is not the case, the strategies are stabilizing poultry meat as an unquestionable human right, both as a source of income for producers and as a direct source of food for consumers.

When the Global Strategy recommends that "comprehensive disease control plans, supported by substantial financial resources to tackle the HPAI problem" should be developed, " country by country in a coordinated manner", it is not up to countries to define "the HPAI problem"; rather, this is already done with the Global Strategy.[151] Therefore, the countries are responsible for finding the most suitable way to handle the problem locally, to control disease *and* to secure poultry production.

Several studies have already challenged the vertical view on global-local connections by demonstrating how "global advice" or "demands from above" may not be implemented due to "local resistance", or they are adjusted to meet

[149] The Global Strategy as well as the Turkish National Strategy is referring to avian influenza as a "complex problem" in general terms (FAO, OIE and WHO 2005 May: 5; 2005Nov: 5; Ivanov, Yanko 2007: 29). They are also emphasising more specific complex relations several places, e.g., the "complex interactions between the avian influenza virus, the hosts and the changing environment" (FAO, OIE and WHO 2005 May: v; 2005 Nov: ix; Ivanov, Yanko 2007: 77) and "the complex interface between farming systems, livestock trade, food safety and public health". (FAO, OIE and WHO 2005 May: v; 2005 Nov: x). Moreover: "The control of HPAI is a multidisciplinary exercise, addressing the complex interactions between technical, institutional, policy, political and socio-economic issues, all of which necessitate engagement of a large number of partners." (FAO, OIE and WHO 2005 May: 21; 2005 Nov: 27).

[150] Latour, Bruno 1990

[151] FAO, OIE and WHO 2005 May: 2; 2005 Nov: 2

"local conditions".[152] By following the connection from the Asian outbreak places, via the Global Strategy – which should not be mistaken for being *The Global*, but rather a locally produced document – to the Turkish National Strategy, I approach the global as *horizontal connections*. Hence, I study the becoming of global issues through processes and relations of *connecting locals*.[153]

By demonstrating how the Asian experience has been inscribed in the Global Strategy in a way that makes the strategy document densely populated by ducks, I have shown how the Asian experience contributed *locally*, that is in the global strategy, in enacting a "global problem". Hence, this "global problem," which has largely been enacted by Asian ducks, moves on to another locality, the Turkish National Strategy, and contributes in re-enacting the Asian duck-problem as a Turkish backyard poultry-problem. This analysis has shown how translocal connections are multilayered, which should not be confused with hierarchical; how they consist of layers of heterogeneous realities – like ponds in ponds. Some realities move; they work and have effect. Others remain; they do not move, but also these have effect; they influence in other ways, through their absence. This way of enacting the global, namely as *connecting locals*, needs further exploration: In the following chapter, I will explore how the detection of HPAI in several European countries contributed to alter the global avian influence threat within the Global Strategy

152 For and overview please refer to Tsuda Takeyuki, Maria Tapias and Xavier Escandell 2014. See also Porter, Natalie 2013b; 2014

153 Law, John and Annemarie Mol 2008; Ong, Aihwa 1999; Strathern, Marilyn 2004; Tsing, Anna 2005

# 5. HPAI (H5N1) spreads to Europe and turns into a wild bird issue

> Since the inception of this [Global Strategy] document in May 2005, avian influenza has progressed from Southeast Asia into Northern China, Mongolia, Kazakhstan, Russia and more recently in Eastern Europe and Turkey, with increasing evidence that the disease is being carried by wild birds migrating along flyways, well beyond the originally infected foci in Southeast and East Asia.
>
> Due to the recent spread of the disease in other regions, the Global Strategy is expanded ( . . . )[1]

Not only did the avian influenza virus progress to new territories, and not only did the Global Strategy expand in number of pages during the few months between the Draft version was published in May 2005 and the Final version was launched in November of the same year – as the above text taken from the Final version shows, recent developments brought wild migratory birds into the strategy documents. In this text, we see how the wild birds' role is being extended: it is not only about "wild birds" anymore, but also about "wild *migratory* birds"; from being reservoirs and sources of local infection, wild birds moving along migratory flyways are becoming major long distance carriers of viruses, in the updated Final version of the Global Strategy.

Bruno Latour explains *inscription* as "[a] general term that refers to all the types of transformations through which an entity becomes materialised into a sign, an archive, a document, a piece of paper, a trace."[2] In order to understand how local events contribute in re-enacting the "global crisis" of avian influenza, this chapter will study the *inscription* of the spread of the virus beyond Asia – to Europe and into the Final version of the Global Strategy. As in the previous chapter, I will also study the connections between the Global Strategy and the Turkish National Strategy.

A central question in this chapter will be: how do inscriptions of new events contribute to move the "global threat" of avian influenza as it is being re-textualized, to paraphrase Kristin Asdal, and hence re-materialized, in the updated version of the Global Strategy? As this introduction has already briefly shown, and as will be thoroughly analysed in this chapter, when the spread of avian influenza from Asia to Europe is inscribed and textualized

1 FAO, OIE, WHO 2005 Nov: vii

2 Latour, Bruno 1999: 306

in the Final version, avian influenza is increasingly becoming a wild bird issue. By bringing along Asdal's relational approach, introduced in the previous chapter, I will remain attentive to how this way of ordering avian influenza as a wild bird issue relates to other ways of ordering avian influenza, studied in the previous chapter. There, my analysis showed how avian influenza was enacted as an issue of emergence, as an economic issue, as a poultry issue and as a human health issue. Related to this, I will also follow up on the relation between what Latour coins as "matters of fact" and "matters of concern". How does the controversial and uncertain role of wild birds as a means for spreading disease fit together with the generally agreed upon certain role of humanly induced mechanisms for spread, such as transportation and trade?

A major outcome of my studies of the strategy documents in the previous chapter relates to how the strategy is ordering the "complex"[3] "global threat"[4] of avian influenza in one particular way. This ordering is not made in isolation. I have argued that the enacted "global threat" did not come into being from nowhere; rather it is a product of joint local efforts, and results from the contributions of individuals, acting for example in the name of UN organs – representatives of the *"world organizations"*. Crucially, they *are* not the world; they are *making* a world; they are enacting*a* reality out of many. In this way, I have already proposed that we should think of the global not as a stable and external entity, but as an ongoing process of *connecting locals*. This approach will be further developed in this chapter. In doing so I will take it a step further and also actively engage with context.

Context has been a recurring problem in STS studies. More recently though, scholars centrally positioned within the field of STS are turning this potentially reductionist, explanatory tool, context, into a tool for open-ended exploration and experimentation. Rather than claiming the context to be decisive for the way issues are being formed, context is itself heterogeneous and a current outcome of on-going processes and relations. Kristin Asdal and Ingunn Moser suggest that, "[i]f context is the problem, then contexting might be an answer".[5] Drawing this recourse into my analysis, context is not simply "background" distinct from the strategy documents, but it is also situations within which these documents were made, *and* situations the making of which they contribute to. Hence, context is not limited to historical past, but is an ac-

3 FAO, OIE, WHO 2005 May: v, 5, 13, 21, Appendix 1; FAO, OIE, WHO 2005 Nov: ix, x, 5, 17, 27, Appendix 1

4 FAO, OIE, WHO 2005 May: iii, 4, 30, 55; FAO, OIE, WHO 2005 Nov: vii, 5, 40, 69

5 Asdal, Kristin and Ingunn Moser 2012: 293

tive part of present situations and the way futures are enabled through these.[6] Building on my analytical approaches from the previous chapter, where I studied how the strategy documents are realizing avian influenza – that is how texts contribute to enact reality in certain ways – I aim to take this one step further in the current chapter and pay attention to how the process of textualizing also involves *contexting*. That is, how the strategy documents are enacting context in the sense of historical past – for example the Draft version – and re-enact contexts for the future. Furthermore, context must also include the situation and process through which I have analysed and made sense of these documents, hence this chapter also offers reflection on that.

As an attempt to practice contexting, I will briefly sketch out, or textualize, a version of the context in which I was reading these strategy documents, and which also partially overlaps with the context in which the National Strategy was written. An overall ambition is to open up, rather than to draw out a singular context that explains why things are as they are. My aim is to show alternatives; that context, like reality, is complex and comes in different versions that either go together or do not. After reflecting on context, I will turn to the Draft version of the Global Strategy where I will study how avian influenza is enacted as a wild bird issue, an issue that was not examined in the previous chapter. The next section will trace how wild birds enter the Final version, before I, in the following section, analyse how wild birds contribute to re-enacting avian influenza as a wild bird issue in the Final Version of the Global Strategy and in the Turkish National Strategy. Especially throughout the latter two parts, I also aim to reflect on what is often thought of as global-local relations, but which I, through my analysis here, will argue is better thought of as *connecting locals*.

## Contextualizing the strategy writing, the reading, and the context of the spread of avian influenza

It is May 2007. I have just recently arrived in Turkey for my first fieldtrip. Among the texts I had been reading back in Norway during the previous months were the two versions of the Global Strategy. As I would see when visiting the office of the AI project in Ankara during this fieldwork, the National Strategy was just in the making. Reading the two versions of the Global Strategy, it all seemed so straightforward. Still, I could not figure out what to

[6] This argument is especially stressed in Asdal's contribution in this special issue of Science Technology and Human Values on Context already referred to; Asdal, Kristin 2012).

make of the documents. I was happy to take a break from the documents, and was eager to return to Turkey, where I had been so many times before. This time would be different; the context of this trip was different, I went there to study avian influenza.

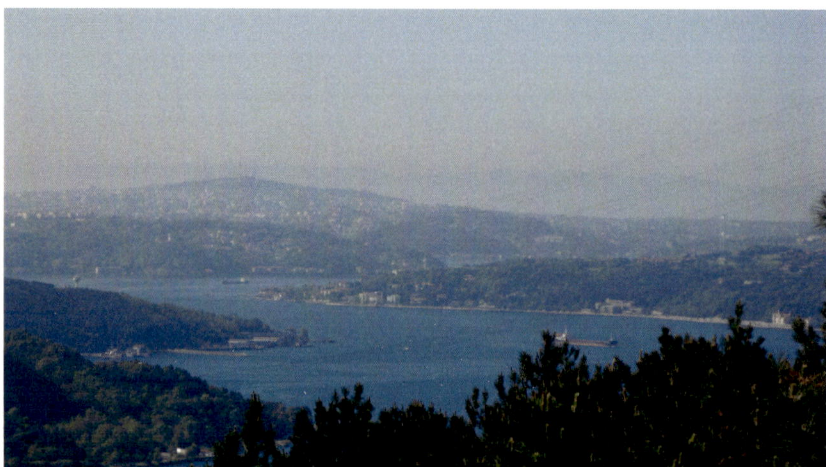

*The Bosporus. Picture from fieldtrip May 2007.*

Down below us the Bosporus is meandering. Large ships are soundlessly floating through the strait on their way between the Black Sea and the Marmara Sea, which leads to the Aegean Sea, the Mediterranean Sea and farther beyond. We have found our way to this marvellous viewpoint not to watch the cargo ships, nor the flowing water. Neither did we care about the heavy traffic crossing the two Bosporus bridges connecting the Asian and the European continents (at the left and right side, respectively, of the Bosporus strait in the picture above). We are here to watch the on-going spring migration as soaring birds are utilizing the air currents of the strait on their journey back north from their southern winter habitats. While working to make appointments with some of the largest poultry producers in the country, positioned close to Bandırma on the Southern side of the Marmara Sea at the southern Mouth of the Bosporus (where we are facing in this picture), I found it worthwhile to use the opportunity to go bird watching with a wild bird enthusiast I was introduced to in Istanbul.[7]

[7] Getting in contact with this bird watcher is mentioned in Chapter 3 as a turning point taking place at an early phase of my first fieldwork. Planned attempts to make contact with various organization turned out to be difficult but coincidence led me to this bird watcher who could

Even though avian influenza is commonly referred to as a poultry disease, the role of wild birds, in particular of wild migratory birds, in long distance spread, had been a hot topic for intense discussions over the last one and a half years, since the highly pathogenic avian influenza caused by the H5N1 virus entered Turkey and other European countries. Hence, in this context, where the role of wild birds were a matter of intense debate, a matter scientific studies,[8] and a matter of practical interventions aimed at separating domestic birds from wildlife, I thought it would be worthwhile spending this sunny Sunday getting a crash course in wild birds' migration on the Bosporus hillsides.

Indeed, during the next months of this fieldtrip, as well as during later fieldtrips, I would find myself in several situations where wild birds would be a central matter of concern. Already a few days after bird watching by the Bosporus, when I met with Turkey's third largest poultry producer, Şeker Piliç, I was surprised to learn that both this and other large companies were raising broilers in integrated farms in Kiziksa, the little village where the first outbreak in Turkey was detected. As I showed in Chapter 3, and as will be further examined in the current chapter, this outbreak was ordered in a way that contributed to making it a wild bird issue, and not an issue of poultry production. When continuing my fieldtrip to Ankara, where I met with the AI project team, wild birds appeared again.[9] The central team member I talked to vividly explained how they thought migratory birds were surprised by a cold wave, and thus brought the virus across the Black Sea to Turkey. A small part of what he told me can be found among the quotes opening this very book. Later on, he sent me to talk to people in Turkey's Bird Research Association, *Kuş Arastırmaları Derneği* (KAD), where I learned, among other things, about the

point out actual and relevant organizations, and he told me about the recently started AI project.

8 A comprehensive overview of the debates on the role of wild birds is outside the scope of this project, but among the many articles and reports that informed my work and which was available or in the making as the H5N1 virus spread to Europe the following should be mentioned: Butler, Declan 2006; Chen et al. 2006; EFSA 13/09/2005; ESFA 12/05/2006; Fear, Chris J. and Maï Yasué 2006; Gilbert, Marius Xiangming Xiao, Joseph Domenech, Juan Lubroth, Vincent Martin and Jan Slingenbergh 2006; Liu, J. et al. 2005; Matthews, Christopher 2006; Normille, Dennis 2005; See also Delany, Simon, Jan Veen and Jacquie Clark (Eds.) 2006; Delany, Brouwer and Veen (Eds.) 2007; Didrickson, Özgür Keşaplı, Özge Keşaplı Can and Can Bilgin 2007; UNEP/CMS 2007; Weber, Thomas P. and Nikolaos I. Stilianakis 2007

9 What I throughout this book refer to as the AI project has previously been introduced as the EU funded *Technical Assistance to Avian Influenza Preparedness and Response Project in Turkey* assigned to assist national authorities in handling avian influenza in the country.

national bird-ringing scheme, and how the Association was involved in avian influenza surveillance in wild birds.

Reading through the Global Strategy after returning from this fieldtrip gave me another grip on the texts. During the fieldtrip, the context within which I read the Draft and the Final versions changed; my experiences influenced my reading. By using the "compare documents" function in Adobe Acrobat Pro I could easily trace the places where text had been changed. Manually comparing the changed areas highlighted by mark-ups in the Final version with the original Draft version shows that the original text remains nearly unchanged, but that new text is added *inscribing* the recent events into the Global Strategy. My immediate impression was that wild birds appeared frequently in the text that was added to the Final version. Was that because I had become oversensitive to wild birds during my fieldwork, or was it because they were playing a bigger role in the Final version?

Inspired by the epidemiologists and ornithologists I met during my fieldtrips to Turkey, I decided to apply their methodology and conduct a wild bird census. While they performed wild bird censuses as part of their epidemiological investigations, in order to record wild bird abundance in areas that have been defined as relevant in relation to avian influenza outbreaks, I conducted my census work within the body text of the two versions of the Global Strategy.[10] Instead of binoculars and telescope, I made use of the find function and advanced search option in Adobe Acrobat Pro. Their findings will be further explored in Chapters 6 and 7 of this volume. My own census resulted in 14 and 77 hits on "wild birds" (or directly related terms) in the Draft and the Final versions respectively.[11] As mentioned in the previous chapter, the total number of pages increased from 64 to 86 pages. Hence, the count sustained my impression of a conspicuous increase in wild bird abundance in the text added to the Final version of the Global Strategy, as compared to the Draft. This also justified my own interest in exploring how avian influenza is enacted as a wild bird issue in these documents; by studying wild birds and the places where they occur within these documents and in the National Strategy I aim to understand what is happening when wild birds are "flocking" into the strategies.

[10] Unless mentioned, appendices and tables are not included in my wild bird census. For examples of census work in outbreak investigations in Turky see e.g. Van den Ende, Rinus and Ragip Bayraktar 2008 Sazkoy; Newman, Scott, Nick Honhold, Javier Sanz-Alvarez and Kiraz Erciyas 2008.

[11] The count covers only the body text (table of content and appendices are not included) and it includes words such as "wild birds", "wild migratory birds", "migratory species", "wild fowl", "wild carriers", "flyways", "(migratory) routes" and "wildlife" (which in nearly all cases refers to avian species).

The Draft version of the Global Strategy was written within a context where avian influenza was currently an on-going problem in Asia, but where further spread within and beyond Asia was a matter of concern. The updated version of the Global Strategy was written within a context where spread beyond Asia – to Europe and possibly further – was currently taking place. As we saw in the previous chapter, humanly induced mechanisms for spread were enacted both as a matter of fact and as a matter of concern in regard to HPAI spread. As my "wild bird census" above shows, the role of migratory birds in long distance spread of HPAI H5N1 is becoming a matter of great concern in this document. Brita Brenna insists that "the book [in her case the first natural history of Norway, written by Erik Pontoppidan in the mid-18th century] is the best guide to its contexts."[12] My preliminary analysis of the text added to the Final version indicates that the concerns related to the role of wild birds in long distance spread was a crucial context when the Global Strategy was updated. Context, though, according to Brenna and the other contributors to the special issue of Science Technology and Human Values on just *Context*, is not only something that influences, or has influence *on*, a book or a text. Rather – and this goes well together with how I, with Asdal, have claimed that texts are making things real; that texts realize – texts also influence their context. In his chapter I therefore aim to follows Brenna's advice to analyse the strategy documents "with an eye on which contexts the book makes for itself". Or more precisely, and in accordance with the research questions posed above, how are the documents re-contextualizing avian influenza as it spreads beyond Asia?[13] How does the inscriptions of the spread beyond Asia contribute to re-enacting avian influenza? How does the wild bird issue go together with the other versions of avian influenza examined in the previous chapter? Moreover, how do wild birds contribute to re-enact the context of safe poultry hold; how are they re-contextualizing how to live securely – biosecurity?

## Wild birds enacting avian influenza in the Draft version of the Global Strategy

Wild birds appear in six different places and are, as noted above, mentioned 14 times within the body text of the Draft version of the Global Strategy. How is avian influenza being enacted as a wild bird issue in these places? That is what I will explore in this section.

12 Brenna, Brita 2012: 359

13 Brenna, Brita 2012: 359. An important point of Brenna's article is to focus on audiences and how they are addressed in the text.

The first place wild birds contribute in the Draft version is in a list of arguments advocating "Why a Global Strategy?".[14] It states that:

- HPAI results from low pathogenic avian influenza (LPAI), which is present in wild birds in many parts of the world. All countries in the world are at risk of being infected unexpectedly.[15]

Further down in the same section we can read that:

The role of wildlife in the spread of avian influenza is still not clearly understood. While the gene pool of the avian influenza viruses is relatively benign in its natural wildlife population hosts, it can evolve rapidly after infecting and adapting to domestic poultry.[16]

In both places, two interconnected binaries are in operation. One is avian influenza viruses, which may be low pathogenic (LPAI) or high pathogenic (HPAI). The second binary is the types of avian species, which in this text are either wild birds or domestic poultry. In this text, wild birds are associated with relatively harmless, low pathogenic avian influenza virus. Lethal, high pathogenic avian influenza virus is assumed to develop within domestic poultry. Still, it is the wild birds that pose the threat in these places in the Draft version of the Global Strategy. This is due to their potential capacity to carry "benign" avian influenza viruses *to* – and here it is crucial to note the direction of viral flow – domestic poultry, in which the viruses may "evolve" and cause severe disease.

In this latter text it is also worth noticing that "[t]he role of wildlife in the spread of avian influenza is still not clearly understood". In this way, the role of wildlife in spread is enacted as uncertain.

In the next three places where wild birds appear in this document, something is happening. Here they are "implicated as reservoirs of disease".[17] In two of these places it is further emphasized "that complete eradication of [HPAI in Asia] will not be possible ( . . . ) due to its presence in wild bird reservoirs."[18] In the subsection titled5.7 *Wildlife reservoirs are a source of HPAI infection,* wild birds' role as reservoirs and as a hindrance for eradication is further stabilized, and here they also obstruct biosecurity measures:

---

[14] FAO, OIE, WHO 2005 May: 2

[15] Op.cit., *bullet and bold types in original*

[16] FAO, OIE, WHO 2005 May: 3; FAO, OIE, WHO 2005 Nov 3; Ivanov, Yanko 2007:77

[17] This quote is from FAO, OIE, WHO 2005 May: 17 and the two other places referred to here are to be found on p. 5 and p. 14.

[18] FAO, OIE, WHO 2005 May: 5, 14

Epidemiological studies suggest that wild birds have likely played a role in the transmission of H5N1 viruses *to* domestic poultry. The capacity of wild birds to carry HPAI H5N1 viruses presents a major difficulty in applying biosecurity measure aiming at the avoidance of contacts between domestic poultry and wild birds. Eradication of the virus to prevent HPAI infection may not be completely achievable in certain farming systems.[19]

Again, the interrelated binaries wild/domestic and low/high pathogenic as well as direction are also crucial when wild birds are enacted as reservoirs, virus transmitters, and obstructers of biosecurity measures and eradication efforts. The direction is the same as in the text examined above; virus transmission is flowing in one direction, from wild to domestic exclusively.

Regarding pathogenicity something is happening, though. Wild birds are no longer associated with benign LPAI viruses only; here they have here turned into sources, transmitters, and carriers of HPAI viruses as well. How this transformation has happened is, as we saw in the previous chapter on avian influenza as an emerging disease, not reflected upon in this strategy. As HPAI viruses are generally assumed to evolve from LPAI within densely populated domestic poultry production systems, it is reasonable to think that, in order for wild birds to become carriers and transmitters of HPAI, there must be flow in the opposite direction too; from domestic to wild. Furthermore, since the flow in that direction causes contamination of wildlife with high pathogenic virus that has evolved within and among domestic poultry, avian influenza could have been enacted as an issue of environmental contamination or as a pollution issue. However, this does not happen.

On the contrary, the Global Strategy is again working with a one-way approach, as it is lists six key issues for applied research. What the Strategy here is calling calls for here is:

? To determine the role of pigs [?!?] and other wild birds in transmission of H5N1 *to* domestic poultry.[20]

In contrast to the certainty regarding the role of human activity in long and short distance spread – as we saw in the previous chapter where emergence came to be about spread to new places – the role of wildlife in transmission

[19] FAO, OIE, WHO 2005 May: 13, *italics added.*

[20] FAO, OIE, WHO 2005 May: 21. I assume that pigs are mentioned here as the more common way of transmission of virus from avian species to humans goes via pigs due to genetic composition. As a remark I can mention that when the list of key issues for research are brought along in the National Strategy this sentence has been divided into two, and pigs are turned into wild pigs: "· To determine the possible role of wild pigs." And "· To elucidate the role of different wild birds species in transmission of H5N1 to domestic poultry in Turkey." (Ivanov, Yanko 2007: 79)

and spread is surrounded by uncertainty.[21] This uncertainty, and the potentially critical implications, motivates the strategy's call for special attention on the role of wild birds, first of all in short distance spread, as migratory birds are only mentioned one time in the body text of the Draft version.

It is in subsection 2.6, titled *Globalized markets have caused HPAI to spread rapidly*, that the uncertain but "possible role of wild migratory birds" is being brought up as a contrast to the certain "danger of international spread of HPAI [which] has increased by the dynamics of regional and international trade and the movement of people"[22]

To sum up the analysis of wild birds in the Draft version, their performance is there both associated with certainty and uncertainty. What is enacted as certain is their role as reservoirs for LPAI, from which HPAI can evolve. That the LPAI virus can turn highly pathogenic is a matter of concern; how this is happening is, as the analysis in the previous chapter showed, not a matter of concern in the body text. Hence, we cannot see, in the body text of the Global Strategy, when and how wild birds are getting the role as source and carrier of HPAI virus. Furthermore, this role does remain surrounded by uncertainty, though it is no less a matter of concern, mainly in relation to local virus transmission and short distance spread. A final remark on the role of wild birds, that I want to keep in mind when moving on to studying wild birds in the body text of the Final version, concerns direction, which we have seen is exclusively *from* wild *to* domestic.

On a list of recommendations from the *OIE/FAO International Scientific Conference on Avian Influenza*, to be found in the appendices, migratory as well as resident birds are enacted as targeted objects for surveillance and epidemiological studies. The wide spread of the virus taking place during the months after the Draft was published provided good opportunities for such real-world studies.

## Strategy revised: Wild birds are flocking in

The number of mentions of wild birds increased to 77 hits in the Final version of the Global Strategy, as compared with 14 in the Draft version. How did this abundance come abut? Wild birds are immediately flocking into the Foreword

21 As we saw, the strategy makes clear that "[t]he danger of international spread of HPAI has increased by the dynamics of regional and international trade and the movement of people." (FAO, OIE, WHO 2005 May: 4)

22 FAO, OIE, WHO 2005 May: 4

of the Final version of the Global Strategy. The original text persists, but the following sentence is added in the Final version:

> Since the inception of this document in May 2005, avian influenza has progressed from Southeast Asia into Northern China, Mongolia, Kazakhstan, Russia and more recently in Eastern Europe and Turkey, with *increasing evidence* that the disease is being carried by wild birds migrating along flyways, well beyond the originally infected foci in Southeast and East Asia.[23]

It is this geographical "progress" of the avian influenza that is taking place during the months between the publishing of the Draft and the completion of the Final version and which is given place, by inserted parts and revisions, in the Final version of the Global Strategy. Already here, in the Foreword, wild *migratory* birds are entering the Strategy. Furthermore, flyways, not explicitly mentioned in the Draft, are efficiently put to work in the Final version as means for HPAI virus to be carried by wild migratory birds, "well beyond the originally infected foci in Southeast and East Asia". Further on, "[a] group of new, non-infected countries" that are characterized as being "at immediate risk", appear to be so due to their location "along the flyways of migratory birds that carry the H5N1 virus".[24]

Domestic ducks, which were playing an important role in the interpretations of outbreaks in Asia, as we saw in the previous chapter, have no place in the overview of newly infected countries added in the Final version. Rather, wild birds are becoming the new, main actors; on the approximately one page presentation of *Newly infected countries in Asia and Europe*, "wild birds" occur 13 times.[25] That is only one occurrence less than in the total body text of the Draft document.

Among the outbreaks that contributed to bringing wild birds into the Final version – those that are enacted as "highly suggestive of the role of wild birds in the epidemiology of HPAI" – are the initial outbreaks in Turkey and Romania.[26] The country reviews tell us that, "[d]eaths due to H5N1 were reported in domestic turkeys in Turkey, and in whooping swans in Romania."[27] The Strategy offers no further reflections on how or why the outbreak among domestic turkeys in Turkey is "highly suggestive of the role of wild birds in the epidemi-

23 FAO, OIE, WHO 2005 Nov: vi,*italics added.* I use the same text in the opening of this chapter.

24 FAO, OIE, WHO 2005 Nov: viii

25 FAO, OIE, WHO 2005 Nov: 10–11. The term *"wild birds" does here also include "wild water fowl", "migratory birds", "whooping swans" and "wildlife".*

26 FAO, OIE, WHO 2005 Nov: 10

27 FAO, OIE, WHO 2005 Nov: 10

ology of HPAI", in other words how this outbreak is turning into a wild bird issue. As we saw in Chapter 3, this work had already been done by the Turkish authorities in their outbreak reports. The way this outbreak was ordered – as a wild bird issue – in the report from the Turkish Ministry of Agriculture and Rural Affairs, keeps its shape when moving into the Global Strategy. Hence, it contributes, together with other outbreaks in other countries, in enacting the "global threat" of avian influenza.

In the Romanian outbreak contributing to the Final version, the whooping swans are acting alone. As I showed above, "[d]eaths due to H5N1 were reported in ( ... ) whooping swans in Romania."[28] Moving to the *Immediate Notification Report,* sent from Romanian national authorities to OIE as soon as the first outbreak was officially detected, the swans are however no longer acting alone. Actually, they are not acting at all; here the reported "Affected Population" is "58 laying hens and 42 ducks in a single backyard farm".[29] This could be explained by the fact that disease in wildlife is not notifiable to the OIE. In the case of H5N1 avian influenza, it still appears to be the practice to also report cases in wildlife, and in relation to this outbreak in Romania, the first wild birds, together with an increasing number of domestic poultry, do occur in the second follow-up report sent a few days later.[30] My aim is not to investigate the outbreak investigations in Romania, but bringing in these reports shows that avian influenza infection could, like in Turkey, just as well have become a domestic poultry issue. Letting the whooping swans act alone by *not* bringing in the domestic hens and ducks from the *Immediate Notification Report*, the Global Strategy is enacting this outbreak, like the mentioned one in Turkey, in such a way that it "may be highly suggestive of the role of wild birds in the epidemiology of HPAI."[31]

Russia, Kazakhstan and Mongolia experienced several outbreaks during the months between the publishing of the Draft and the Final versions, and are subsequently given more attention. Despite that "[c]onclusive evidence for

28 FAO, OIE, WHO 2005 Nov: 10

29 OIE Wahid Immediate notification report received 07.05.2005 from Mr Gabriel Predoi, , Direction générale sanitaire vétérinaire, Directeur général, Bucarest, Romania http://www.oie.int/wahis_2/public/wahid.php/Reviewreport/Review?reportid=5189, *last read 26.03.2014*

30 OIE Wahid, Follow-up Report No 2, date of report 14.10.2005 http://www.oie.int/wahis_2/public/wahid.php/Reviewreport/Review?reportid=5204, *last read 26.03.2014*

"Source of Infection" is determined to be "Contact with wild Species." No further specifications or identifications are provided in this report, and as I will come back to in the next chapter on outbreak investigation "contact with wild species" may work as a conclusion when other sources are not found.

31 FAO, OIE, WHO 2005 NOV: ix, also cited above

the involvement of wild birds in the introduction of H5N1 virus does not exist", neither for the cases in Russia nor in the other countries, "several factors strongly indicate a potential role for wild birds in the spread of infection."[32]

The inscriptions of these recent events are providing "increasing evidence" of the role of migratory birds in long distance spread. Thus, on the list of "key reasons" explaining "rationale for developing and implementing a global strategy for the control of HPAI", the following point is added in the final version: "?gHPAI may be transported widely and quickly by migratory birds, along flyways and in resting or nesting areas."[33] A "may" does still indicate an amount of uncertainty. However, it is more likely than that it *might* happen, and most importantly, it is likely enough to be added to the list of key reasons legitimizing the Strategy.

By studying how avian influenza is spreading to Europe from Asia, as this move is enacted in the Final version of the Global Strategy, I have now shown how migratory flyways are taking over for highways, railways, air(plane)ways and seaways; responsibility for spread, also over long distances, is being reassigned from humans to wild birds. In this way, the responsibility for spread – the mechanisms and means that are enabling worldwide mobility for virus – is distributed beyond human activities.

This shift to flyways and migratory birds contributes to the re-ordering of avian influenza. As my analyses have shown so far, a version of the wild bird issue made wild birds responsible for spread, and this version finds its way into the Final version of the Global Strategy. In other words, wild birds are not only enacted in a way that make them able to transport viruses over long distances, they also contribute in moving the strategy; to *re-place* the target for interventions from the domestic to the wild.

## Wild birds perform in the Final version of the Global Strategy and in the Turkish National Strategy

How do wild birds contribute to re-enacting avian influenza as its spread to Europe is inscribed in the Final version of the Global Strategy? Moreover, how is avian influenza enacted as a wild bird issue in the Turkish National Strategy? As these documents work as relational spaces where heterogeneous avian influenza issues are co-existing, how does avian influenza as a wild bird issue go together with other versions of avian influenza within and between the different documents? These are the matters of concern in this section.

32 FAO, OIE, WHO 2005 NOV: 10–11

33 FAO, OIE, WHO 2005 Nov: 2

## Uncertainty is getting less uncertain

"The role of wildlife in the spread of avian influenza is still not clearly understood," we could read when studying the Draft version of the Global Strategy above.[34] In the Final version, this sentence is extended by these words: "but seems to be increasingly important".[35] The full sentence in the Final version of the Global Strategy has also found its way into the National Strategy. Above, we saw how the initial outbreak in Turkey contributed to enacting the "global" avian influenza problem as a wild bird issue. As this sentence is copied from the Global Strategy and passed on to the National Strategy, this version is travelling back to Turkey; it is a matter of concern moving between Turkey and the Global Strategy in a way that contributes to stabilizing "[t]he role of wildlife in the spread of avian influenza [as something that] is still not clearly understood, but seems to be increasingly important."[36]

The role of wild birds is also strengthened by other small but powerful reformulations. For example, "[e]pidemiological *studies* suggest that wild birds [only] likely played a role in the transmission of H5N1 to domestic poultry" in the Draft version; this is turned into "[e]pidemiological *observations* suggest that wild birds *very* likely played a role" in the Final version.[37] In addition to these adjustments of this sentence, which opens the subsection titled *Wildlife reservoirs are a source of HPAI infection*, the text has expanded to more than the double of the original length, as the following is added to this section in the Final version:

> There is *increasing evidence* that the introduction of H5N1 from Southeast and East Asia to other regions *may* have been due to migratory wild birds from which H5N1 was isolated, and *could* have died from the disease along their migratory routes. However, some findings also *suggest* that H5N1 viruses *could* have been transmitted between migratory birds. The introduction of HPAI to other parts of Asia *may* indicate that some migratory bird species act as carriers, and can transport HPAI over longer distances. Short-distance transmission between farms, villages or contaminated local water bodies is likewise *a distinct possibility*.[38]

"[I]ncreasing evidence" is, in this text, accompanied by uncertainty of the actual role of migratory birds in long distance spread. The uncertainty is enacted by all the "mays" and "coulds", and by "suggesting", and as a "distinct pos-

34 FAO, OIE, WHO 2005 May: 3

35 FAO, OIE, WHO 2005 Nov: 3

36 Ivanov, Yanko 2007:77; FAO, OIE, WHO 2005 Nov: 3

37 FAO, OIE, WHO 2005 May: 13, *italics added*; FAO, OIE, WHO 2005Nov: 17, *italics added*.

38 FAO, OIE, WHI 2005 Nov: 17; Ivanov, Yanko 2007: 40

sibility", all emphasised by me in the text above by using italics. In this way, "increasing evidence", "observations" and "increasing [...] importance" is accompanied with a certain amount of modest uncertainty as wild birds find their way into the Final version of the global strategy.

At the same time as the uncertainty regarding the actual role of wild birds in long distance spread is acknowledged in the latter text, which can be found both in the Final version of the Global Strategy and in the National Strategy above, no other possibilities interfere with this theory as presented. This might not be strange, as this section, according to its heading, is dedicated "*Wildlife reservoirs* [that]*are a source of HPAI infection*". However, in the section of the Global Strategy titled*Globalized markets have caused HPAI to spread rapidly*, which apparently is about domestic and commercial aspects, the following sentence suddenly occurs, reminding us that "[t]he possible role of wild migratory birds is not yet fully elucidated."[39] While wild birds are given an opening when domestic and commercial issues are discussed, the opposite inference does not take place. This section focuses exclusively on wild birds.[40]

In the National Strategy however, in a related section not found in the Global Strategy, titled *Migration of wild birds,* it is mentioned that, "[i]n addition [to wild birds], informal domestic poultry trade within the country may also contribute to the dispersal or spread of HPAI; both wild bird migration and live bird trade need to be assessed and monitored."[41] However, it is only the first option that is discussed further; while wild bird surveillance is given thorough attention, no further concern is paid to how, or where or by whom informal trade can be targeted, neither in this section nor other places in the Turkish National Strategy. Furthermore, formal trade is not explicitly mentioned at all.

So far I have traced how small textual changes contribute to making things more certain, but also how the text that is added is, at least in some incidents, enacting a modest uncertainty. In this regard, it is interesting to see how the same outbreaks are enacted as more or as less certain as they appear at various places within the same document. In the *Executive summary*, "[t]hese recent outbreaks*may be suggestive* of the role of wild birds in the epidemiology of HPAI."[42] When the same sentence occurs further on in the document, the same

[39] FAO, OIE, WHO 2005 May: 4; FAO, OIE, WHO 2005 Nov: 4

[40] For a similar argument on how making of absence and presence contribute in "disarciculating alternatives" see Moser 2008

[41] This section cannot be found in the Global Strategy, but major parts of the text is identical with the African Strategy (FAO/ECTAD 2006)

[42] FAO, OIE, WHI 2005 Nov: ix, *italics added*

outbreaks "are *highly suggestive* of the role of wild birds".[43] This illustrates not only how text contributes to making things real, but also how textual nuances contribute to enacting reality in certain, or even quite different, ways.

In the Final version, compared with the Draft, the role of wild birds is stabilized, not by replacing the uncertainty surrounding it in the Draft version with certainty, but by *adding probabilities*. As no text from the Draft version was removed when it was revised and the Final version was completed, the uncertainty reflected at some of these textual places remains. However, the inscription of the recent, wide-reaching spread challenges the uncertainty, not by adding "facts", but by adding a specific set of observations that works alongside the wild bird theories. In other words, no final, clear evidence is reported to have been found; the sum of events however, destabilizes the uncertainty. The story of avian influenza as a wild bird issue is relying on theories of spread and is dependent on having a narrow focus on persistence and spread, limited to wild birds – and not including alternative mechanisms of spread – in order to perform the move from uncertain to less uncertain.[44] In this way, the document is engaging one specific context where wild birds are prominent, and contributes to reinforcing or strengthening this. In other words, a context of the historical past is contributing to enacting the context of the strategies for future actions.[45]

## New spaces I: Emerging topology of risk

> It seems that the virus has moved north and westward along the wildfowl flyway and has spread to domestic poultry whenever there is a chance because of weak biosecurity level of some farms and smallholders. (... ) Since wild birds are difficult to control, the major emphasis must be given on enhancing biosecurity at smallholder level and promoting people's awareness.[46]

This text, added to the final version of the Global Strategy, is enacting a simple topographical model for virus spread where wild birds' flyways or migratory routes is the (*only*) inscribed infrastructure that is enabling viral movement *to* Europe. But, this text is also contributing to an emerging topology of bio*in*security, I will argue; Wild birds are, in this text, explicitly stated to be "difficult to control". Moreover, as they serve as virus reservoirs and sources

[43] FAO, OIE, WHI 2005 Nov: 10, *italics added*

[44] On how realities are co-existing and how they are being made more real or less real in processes of making absence and presence I here draw in particular on Moser, Ingunn (2008)

[45] Asdal, Kristin 2012. See also Asdal, Kristin 2014

[46] FAO, OIE, WHO 2005 Nov: 57 (Appendix 6)

of infection, the kinds of places lying along "wildfowl flyways", are associated with wild birds possibly carrying contaminated baggage from outside. Hence, they represent areas at risk of infection.[47] Further on, in addition to "flyways" and "migratory [bird] routes", other wildlife habitats are entering the Global Strategy with the updates of the Final version. The Final version is, for example, providing space for "resting and nesting areas"[48], "wetlands, rivers, and shorelines" and "streams"[49]. These textualized sites are enacting certain kinds of places where migratory birds, loaded with viral luggage, seek transit or seasonal habitat; hence they become sites where migratory birds might interact with local populations and infect local birds and domestic poultry.

The focus on wild birds is carried forward to the National Strategy where it is emphasised that "Turkey is one of the richest countries for wild bird habitats in Europe and the Middle East with 135 major sites."[50] The strong relation between the country and wild birds is further emphasised by a map, which is the only illustration in the whole document. The map brings Turkey's wetlands and bird habitats protected under the Ramsar Convention into the Strategy. In this way, the map contributes to enacting Turkey as a melting pot for wild birds and avian influenza virus. Below the map, the section continues:

> [Turkey] is situated on four important bird migration routes between Europe, the Middle East, the wider Caspian Sea area and Africa. Lake Manyas, a nature conservation area and renowned stop-over for waterfowl, lies on one route, and the first AI outbreak in the country occurred in free-range turkeys near the lake. This illustrates the threat of AI in wild birds to domestic poultry, and the challenge it poses for control and eradication efforts."[51]

This way of enacting Turkey's geographical position as dominated by wild birds' flyways – and no other potential routes of virus transportation – works efficiently to explain the initial outbreaks that were reported in the country, and contributes with "increasing evidence" to strengthening the wild bird spread theories.[52]

As I showed in Chapter 3, by also mentioning that this province is dominated by intensive poultry production, and that the mentioned Lake Manyas is

---

47 The latter, that wild birds might serve as reservoirs and source of infection, is only implicit in the text quoted here, but as I have shown this is explicitly established concerns other places in these documents.

48 FAO, OIE, WHO 2005 Nov: 2

49 FAO, OIE, WHO 2005 Nov: 13

50 Ivanov, Yanko 2007: 26

51 Ivanov, Yanko 2007: 26

52 FAO, OIE, WHO 2005 Nov: vi, 17; Ivanov, Yanko 2007: 40

literally surrounded by two of the largest poultry producers in Turkey, their integrated broiler farms, layer facilities, feed mills, slaughter houses, local workforce and so on, the text would not only have enacted a different context. It would also have disturbed the clear image of wild migratory birds as the *only* possible transporter of avian influenza to Turkey. This does not happen, however; the large-scale poultry production is not mentioned, and the textualization of migratory flyways and the Ramsar map remain undisturbed in their contribution to strengthening the role of wild birds in the spread of avian influenza to Turkey.

In this way, flyways and associated on-ground habitats are not only working as *the* exclusive network for virus transportation, they are also contributing to enact a particular scenery – *a* topology of high risk areas. The Global Strategy is bringing in "shorelines", "rivers" and "streams" as potentially insecure places in general. The National Strategy is using text and maps to point out such sites on specific spots on the ground. Hence, when the general terms enacting various wild bird habitats in the Global Strategy move to the Turkish Strategy, they are turning into particular places. They are becoming "more real" but also more risky; they are both examples of the kinds of places pointed out as risk areas in the Global Strategy. But at the same time it is the inscription of avian influenza outbreaks in Turkey, among other countries, that have contributed to increasing the importance of wild bird habitats in the Global Strategy. In this way, I will argue that particular outbreak places "on the ground" and general risk sites enacted in the Global Strategy are reinforcing each other, and that they together contribute to enact a specific topology of bio*in*security. Importantly, this topology is dependent on the absence of alternative means of spread other than wild birds that would bring in complexity, and hence make the topology less clear.

That there are no signs of alternative means of virus introduction in the wild bird habitats enacted in the strategy documents does not mean that wild birds exist in isolation. Wetlands, rivers and shorelines do not only provide ground for wild birds to land, but are also access points where viruses may enter *into* local domestic life. By close and attentive reading, we can trace the vague, though vital, connection from migratory wild birds *to* domestic poultry, possibly via local birds; as the Global Strategy emphasises, migratory birds "may transmit the disease to local wild birds, and from there to domestic poultry."[53]

[53] FAO, OIE, WHO 2005 Nov: 13. On "vital connections" I am drawing on Sarah Whatmore 2006.

The one-way direction of virus flow, from wild *to* domestic, which was already set in motion in the Draft version of the Global Strategy, is gaining increasing power with the inscriptions of recent events in the Final version. It gains power as the several incidents of spread are reported, and as these incidents are all being inscribed in the Final version in a way that is enacting them as wild bird issues – exclusively. This has effect in two interrelated ways: Firstly, it strengthens the position of wild bird theories for spread. Secondly, as the role of wild birds in spread is becoming predominant to alternative mechanisms for spread, the latter receives no attention in the text inscribing the avian influenza spread to Europe, and it therefore appears to lose its importance. As shown in the section above, the uncertain role of wild birds in long distance spread is becoming the only possibility, as the alternative of humanly induced mechanisms for spread are being disarticulated with the text added to the Final version.[54]

The way recent outbreaks are inscribed in the strategies, and hence the way they contribute to enact a certain topology of bio*in*security, goes well together with the ways avian influenza was initially enacted as heterogeneous issues in the Draft version of the Global Strategy. For example, when studying the table classifying different poultry production systems, we saw that the level of biosecurity was related to contact with wildlife, and not to contacts through market relations. Furthermore, when studying avian influenza as an emerging disease issue in the previous chapter, we saw that origin was not a matter of concern in these documents. Rather, in the Draft version, it was about the spread of something that was already present. By enacting the means for virus spread to Europe exclusively as a matter of wild birds, avian influenza is being further disconnected from the matter of origin, and it also contributes to making humanly induced mechanisms for spread less important.

In this way, "the intra-actions that make disease a possibility in the first place" is getting even more distant as the spread to Europe is inscribed in the Final version of the Global Strategy.[55] It is exactly this that Steve Hinchliffe, John Allen, Stephanie Lavau, Nick Bingham and Simon Carter are warning against when they give a call in unison for a move from topographic to topologic understanding of disease. Hinchliffe et al. emphasise the shortcomings of what they call a "simple geometrical re-telling of the spread of networked disease" which does not take into account that pathogens are continuously changing; they mutate, drift and reassort as they move between adjacent bodies as

[54] As above I owe much to Ingunn Moser (2008) for the notion of *disarticulating alternatives*, and her analytical approach in regards to the consequences thereof.

[55] Hinchliffe, Steve, John Allen, Stephanie Lavau, Nick Bingham and Simon Carter 2012

well as between continents. What Hinchliffe et al. are drawing attention to is the "relational understanding of disease" and the "entangled interplay of environments, hosts, pathogens and humans." What my analysis has shown, and which these authors would apparently agree to, is that a move to topology has to be inclusive; it must allow complexity, and reflect upon and accept its own incompleteness.[56] By drawing in other contexts, and hence enacting the Turkish outbreak place also as an agro-industrial area with widespread connections *in and out* – for example, highways, railways and harbours, and not exclusively wildfowl flyways – the strategy would be better prepared for the unpredictable future, but perhaps enact a less manageable matter of concern.

## New spaces II: Making space for wildlife experts and ornithologists

The increased focus on wildlife, and in particular wild migratory birds, also sends out a call for a special form of expertise, and thus prepares the ground for certain scientific fields. In the Final version of the Global Strategy *wildlife organisations* enter, and so do "wildlife specialists" and "ornithologists":[57]

> A newly emerging research topic is the role of migratory wild birds in contributing to the spread of HPAI. Monitoring, sampling and analysis of the viral subtypes of avian influenza found in wild birds need to be done in order to fully understand their role in the propagation and spread of highly pathogenic avian influenza viruses. A multidisciplinary approach is required that brings together the competencies of veterinarians, wildlife specialists, ornithologists, virologists, molecular biologists and other resource avenues.[58]

This text also calls for other forms of expertise. "A multidisciplinary approach" is "required", but it is the need to find out about "the role of migratory wild birds" that is making this expertise relevant.[59]

In the National Strategy, only one NGO is mentioned by name. Turkish Bird Research Society appears in the section emphasising the importance of cooperation with international and volunteer organizations. According to the Strategy, this organization "undertook pilot surveillance at three locations in 2006/7 and produced a report: 'Identifying the role of wild birds as a vector and transmitter of Avian Influenza in Turkey (pilot study).'"[60] The results of

56 For one of many contributions reflecting upon how reality is an ongoing process see Law 2004a

57 "wildlife organisations" pp. ix and x; "wildlife specialists" p. 26; "ornithologists" p. 26

58 FAO, OIE, WHO 2005 Nov: 26 The quoted part in whole was added in the Final version and is not to be found in the Draft version.

59 Virologists could also be found in Appendix 5, which was present in both versions.

60 Ivanov, Yanko 2007: 14; Didrickson, Özgür Keşaplı, Özge Keşaplı Can and Can Bilgin 2007

this study are not explicitly mentioned, but in the section titled *Migration of wild birds* it is most likely this study being referred to. In this section, we are given to read that:

[t]he fact that recent studies failed to detect H5N1 HPAI viruses in migrating wild birds in Turkey should not lead to complacency. Since wild bird infections could be much focused, the negative results of initial investigations could have been due to the limited number of surveys undertaken, small sample size, or inadequate timing of such sampling.[61]

Here we encounter several implications of the way wild birds are *the* (apparently only) research issue. The aim was to determine "the role of wild birds as a vector and transmitter" – and no other potential vectors and transmitters were investigated. Neither was it an alternative to find out that wild birds have no or a very limited role.[62] Lack of findings is seen as a matter of methodological weaknesses or limitations; it says something about the methods, but nothing about the object of study or the matter of concern.

In a rather interesting way, the National Strategy is contrasting "uncontrolled importation of live birds" and "the role of wild birds" as matter of assessment and investigation related to "introduction of HPAI virus to Turkey":[63]

The risk of introducing the virus through uncontrolled importation of live birds is almost impossible to assess. The role of wild birds in the introduction of HPAI virus to Turkey, dissemination within the country and their ability to constitute a permanent reservoir of infection is still undetermined.[64]

This text is enacting a wide variety of wildlife activity, including countrywide "dissemination", as more controllable, in the sense of assessable, than a particular human activity, the *illegal* "importation of live birds". The latter is referred to in the text as "uncontrollable". The strategy contributes to fortify the uncontrollable nature of "uncontrollable importation of live birds"; the strategy document does not suggest that the role of this means for spread should be assessed, determined nor controlled; to the contrary, it makes it clear that any such attempt would be futile as the role of "uncontrolled importation" of wild birds for virus introduction "is almost impossible to assess". In regards to wild birds, on the other hand, their role in "introduction" and "dissemination"

61 Ivanov, Yanko 2007: 65, consulting the report from the mentioned pilot study directly, the result coincide; there too no HPAI H5N1 is identified in any of the sampled birds. Didrickson, Özgür Keşaplı, Özge Keşaplı Can and Can Bilgin 2007

62 Ivanov, Yanko 2007: 14

63 Ivanov, Yanko 2007: 66

64 *Op. cit.*

and as a "permanent reservoir" is characterised as "*still* undetermined".[65] Thus, the strategy document projects expectations of "determining" the role of wild birds, which then appears controllable.

Even though it is not being enacted as a matter of research concern, increased biosecurity measures aimed at preventing HPAI entering *into* domestic holdings is frequently mentioned as necessary, in both the Global and the National Strategy. The possibilities and implications of HPAI exiting domestic holdings and going*out* into the wild, for example with contaminated manure, are however not raised as a matter of concern in general, nor as a matter of research in any of the strategy documents.

By studying the text inscribing the spread of HPAI virus beyond Asia in the Global Strategy, and the related National Strategy, it has been possible to trace how uncertainty is becoming less uncertain. Not by bringing in evidence, but by disarticulating alternatives, alternatives that exist as matters of fact, but which are no more matters of concern when the avian influenza spread to Europe is textualized in the Final version of the Global Strategy. Furthermore, we have seen how particular kinds of places – wild bird habitats and flyways – enact sites of bio*in*security accommodating unidirectional virus flow from wild to domestic. Finally, I have shown how the strategies are making wildlife experts and ornithologists the relevant kinds of expertise to consult. Wild birds, their flyways and habitats, and their uncertain though possible role in long distance spread of HPAI viruses contribute to making these forms of expertise relevant. At the same time, wildlife experts and ornithologists are expected to produce knowledge that can reinforce wild birds, flyways and habitats as matters of bio*in*security concerns. In other words, places such as wild bird habitats and people such as scientists and experts are strengthening each other; they are making each other relevant, and they contribute together to enacting a particular topology of bio*in*security.

## Connecting locals

Birdwatching on the Bosporus hillside was peaceful and relaxing. The silence was striking; a remarkable contrast to the Istanbul cacophony of urban life – seagulls included, but honking taxies and shouting street vendors slightly more dominating. When a buzzard occasionally rose up from the forest below us, I became aware of a light rustling sound. Did it come from the soaring bird? Or was it the Black Sea breeze in accompaniment with the pine trees that quietly

65 *Op. cit. italics added*

orchestrated the whispering sound? Or was it the sound of the glittering silver-blue stream of water floating through Bosporus that reached all the way up here? The metropolitan city life below us was going on as normal, but here it became remote; it faded into and with the panoramic view. On the other hand, the birds high up above us came close. As we followed their moves through the binoculars, the soaring birds became our immediate present. They were all that mattered up here; undisturbed, we could follow the birds on their journey towards their northern summer habitats.

As I wrote in the introduction to this volume, when choosing to focus on Turkey in my study of the "global" avian influenza issue, wild birds and migratory birds' flyways were the least important reason to focus on Turkey. Rather, I expected other features of the country, of which several can be viewed from this spot on the Bosporus hillside, to be far more relevant and important. Seeing people and goods moving between the two continents, by ships on the Bosporus and across the Bosporus bridges, it is so very apparent that Turkey in general and Istanbul in particular are working as a "bridge between Asia and Europe". It was this long-deserved characterization, pointing at intercontinental relations that have been going on since at least the times of the Silk Road, together with the large and complex poultry sector, and, at that time of writing my project outline, countrywide outbreaks of HPAI H5N1, that made me assume that Turkey would be a strategic country for my study. Or, to put it in the terms that I have been trained to use during years of interacting with particular analytical approaches and empirical materials, I expected this country and its intra- and inter-national connections to provide a *heterogeneous context* for studying avian influenza.

As my analyses in these two latter chapters have shown, trade or movement of people and goods are, in both versions of the Global Strategy, as well as in the National Strategy for Turkey, enacted as certain and crucial mechanisms for spread. "The role of wildlife in the spread" is however, especially in the Draft version of the Global Strategy, uncertain; it is "still not clearly understood", but already in that document it is a matter of concern.[66] Based on this, wild birds do not achieve their predominant positions in these documents due to successful production of clear evidence and facts; to the contrary, it is the *lack* of evidence that is making them *the* matter of concern.

[66] FAO, OIE, WHO 2005 May: 3. As mentioned in the above analysis, in the final version this sentence has been extended: "The role of wildlife in the spread of avian influenza is still not clearly understood, *but seems to be increasingly important*." (FAO, OIE, WHO 2005: 3, *italics added*) The full sentence is also at work in the National Strategy (Ivanov, Yanko 2007: 77)

The avian influenza spread beyond Asia to Europe provided an opportunity to find out more about this unknown means for spread; a real-life event was taking place. Until then, isolation of a virus from wild, thereby migratory, species had mainly been done from wild birds found in areas adjacent to domestic outbreaks and the epidemiological relation between domestic and wild birds remained unclear. Also, experimental trials had succeeded to produce evidence that wild migratory species could be infected by the HPAI H5N1 virus.[67] Several aspects of these studies were criticised, though. Especially contested were the relevance of laboratory experiments on migratory species, kept under laboratory conditions, and the validity of the data in saying anything about the practical ability of birds to actually, outside laboratories, transport viruses over long distances during migration.[68] But, as Science correspondent Dennis Normille put it in the October 2005 issue of the journal: "As H5N1 reaches Europe, scientists debate the role of wild birds but agree on the need for greater surveillance."[69] While there is no doubt that human movement of contaminated poultry or poultry products can cause avian influenza spread, it is becoming increasingly important to find out *if* and *how* wild birds are playing a role in the spread of HPAI.

It is within this heterogeneous context of wild birds and humanly induced mechanisms for spread, among other issues, that the text inscribing the spread to Europe is contributing to the re-ordering of the "global threat" of HPAI. It is in this context of certainty and uncertainty that wild birds are becoming *the* issue and *the* matter of concern in the text inserted into the Final version. From this, it also follows that context is neither decisive nor explanatory; what is happening is not determined by its context – other issues were also part of this context and could have become *the* issue or *an* issue in the new text, but did not.

Context does *not explain why* wild bird theories are becoming predominant and strengthened, but context is *enabling* it.[70] Paying attention to how various versions of context are co-existing and working together is helping us to understand *how* some issues, and versions thereof – in this case versions of the wild birds issue – are being strengthened and thus enabling the emergence of issues and situations for the future.[71] In this way, I have been drawing on Kristin As-

67 See e.g. Chen, H. et al. 2006

68 See e.g. Fear, Chris J. and Maï Yasué 2006; Weber, Thomas P. and Nikolaos I. Stilianakis 2007; Normille, Dennis 2005.

69 Normille, Dennis 2005: 426

70 Asdal, Kristin 2012: 379

71 *Op. cit.*

dal's argument that enactments of future realities should be seen in relation to, but not as a necessary or as the only possible consequence of, the historical past – the context. How is the growing concern in regard to the wild bird issue affecting other issues related to spread? In other words, what is happening to other parts of the context?

As I have shown, the text already present in the Draft version where it was enacting other matters of concern was not adjusted in the updated version. Importantly though, remaining the same does not necessarily imply that it is not becoming different. To the contrary, I have argued that in this case, what remains the same is, just by remaining the same, also being changed; it is "lagging behind". By massively increasing the number of wild bird mentions – creating an abundance – with the text added in the Final version, and by keeping the original text where other issues were also enacted unchanged, I have argued these latter *alternatives are being disarticulated*, using the words of Moser.[72]

Studying the text inscribing the avian influenza spread to Europe during the summer and autumn months of 2005 resembles my experience on the Bosporus hillside in several ways. On the Bosporus hillside, as in the Final version of the Global Strategy, wild birds are becoming present; their role is becoming real, though still uncertain. It was uncertain which role migratory birds would have in my work and their role in relation to the spread of HPAI virus was (and still is) uncertain. Furthermore, similar to how the complex city life of Istanbul is going on as normal and yet at the same time still feels remote and distant, if not absent, from this spot, also in the strategy document other issues and other means of virus transportation persist; they remain the same, since no text is added or removed, still they are becoming less present. Up here on the hillside, as in the text inscribing the spread, wild birds are all that matters; undisturbed, migratory birds are enacting a particular reality.

But, what are the effects of the reality wild birds are enacting in the Final version of the Global Strategy and in the National Strategy? How do wild birds interfere with matters of bio*in*security? The concern is risk of spread, or more precisely risk of introduction. As we saw in Chapter 3, avian influenza is becoming just as much a matter of bio*in*security as a matter of biosecurity; it is becoming a matter of life that threatens life, and wildlife is enacted as a threat towards domestic life. This leads to my second and third point, which are interrelated, and previously stressed by Hinchliffe et al.: that virus flow is being enacted as going in one direction, without taking into consideration

[72] Moser Ingunn 2008

the complex, flexible or intra-active properties of pathogens.[73] As my analysis in the previous chapter showed, the strategies are enacting viruses as already highly pathogenic: they are not about origin or the processes that enables high pathogenic virus strains to emerge in the first place; here it is spread that matters. When high pathogenic avian influenza spreads to Europe and wild birds are being enacted as the transporters, they are no longer only the source of low pathogenic virus that may develop – reassort or mutate – into high pathogenic virus within domestic conditions; they are enacted as the source or host of HPAI virus. Hence, the role of poultry farms as *virus hatchers* is getting even less important.[74] In these strategy documents, HPAI is enacted as something that *enters into* poultry farms, not as something resulting from them. This contributes to enacting specific kinds of spaces as biosecure. And that will be my fourth point: the biosecurity spaces that are being enacted through these documents are those that are closed; places where the domestic is separated from the wild.

In Turkey, this way of enacting biosecure and bio*in*secure ways of poultry holdings worked, for example, to initiate plans to re-arrange backyard poultry hold in villages in certain parts of the country. The idea was to organise cooperatives where families could – or should, since this was supposed to be obligatory – keep their poultry together in closed, joint poultry houses. In practice, this would mean that instead of having several small flocks of 5 to 30 free-ranging or semi-closed scavenging hens, and possibly a smaller number of other poultry species kept in and around private gardens, larger poultry houses were supposed to be built to provide biosecure housing, and thus protect domestic backyard poultry from potential wild sources of HPAI. A survey measuring the attitudes related to these joint farming plans concluded that massive resistance among the public contributed to preventing the realization of these plans.[75]

Seen in relation to what my analysis in these two chapters shows, these plans to reorganise backyard poultry holdings into joint housing or cooperatives particularly demonstrates three crucial implications of enacting spread as a wild bird issue, in the way it is being done through these strategy documents and their inscription of the spread. Firstly, it demonstrates that wildlife is enacted as *the* major threat, from which domestic life can be secured by walls and

---

[73] Hinchliffe, Steve, John Allen, Stephanie Lavau, Nick Bingham and Simon Carter 2012:

[74] I am here drawing on terms posed by Michael Greger (2006) in the title of his book on avian influenza; *Bird Flu: A Virus of Our Own Hatching.*

[75] Durutan, Nedret and Cüneyt Okan 2006; Sipahi, Cevat., Cengiz. Yalcin, Yavuz Cevger, Yilmaz Aral and L. Genc 2011

physical boundaries. Secondly, it demonstrates how HPAI is being detached from the matter of origin, in that poultry houses are enacted as biosecure, rather than as a place where benign low pathogenic avian influenza viruses can turn highly pathogenic. Thirdly, spread is being enacted as going in one direction; *into* the domestic.

In 2008, FAO, in cooperation with OIE and World Bank (WB), published a paper on biosecurity, *Biosecurity for highly pathogenic avian influenza. Issues and options*, where just such attempts to create biosecure conditions for poultry were being problematized and re-enacted as potentially bio*in*secure. Here, scavenging flocks are enacted as probably of "lower risk of exposure to infection" than commercial flocks, despite this practice of poultry hold involving contact with wildlife.[76] Furthermore, it is suggested that "the consequences of infection may be less in terms of onward spread than for commercial producers because of smaller flock sizes and fewer links to intermediaries, service providers and LBMs [live-bird markets]."[77] Here, other mechanisms for introduction and spread also contribute to enacting secure and insecure poultry practices. Moreover, implicitly, virus flow is enacted as going in two directions at least. My analyses show that the different ways that past events of avian influenza spread to Europe are being enacted contribute to pointing out ways of living with poultry and viruses – as secure and insecure – in the future. At the same time, my analyses also show how spread could have been enacted differently, something which would have pointed out other directions for secure living.

Re-thinking *context* in the context of time, as Asdal encourages us to do – to think of the historical past, of the present that is the history of tomorrow, and of the "future of the past" – may also serve as a useful tool to think about place. Studying the *Global* Strategy in this chapter has drawn attention to how "the *global* avian influenza threat" is actually bits and pieces of locally ordered versions of reality, or bits and pieces of local context. Furthermore, reality, or context, is multiple and layered; some layers or versions are made mobile and travel, others do not, or they travel in another direction. For example, by bringing in the Immediate Notification Reports sent from national authorities to OIE I have shown how both a wild bird version and a domestic bird version of avian influenza travelled from Romania to OIE's offices in Geneva, but that only one of these versions found its way to the Global Strategy. In the case of Turkey, in the version that travelled to the Global Strategy, the affected flock

[76] FAO 2008:49

[77] *Op. cit*

of 1,800 turkeys were enacted as victims of virus introduction from wild birds, and the site they were kept at was enacted as wetlands, wild bird habitat and associated with migratory flyways. The nearby broiler farms remained at the outbreak places. So did additional facilities related to poultry industry as well as all other ways of passage.

Two things can be drawn from this latter point: it shows how what claims to be global, the Global Strategy as well as "the global threat" of avian influenza, consists of bits and pieces of the local. Furthermore, writing and producing this Global Strategy and thus enacting avian influenza as a global threat, is also the outcome of local process carried out by individuals making up particular working groups within and among these "global" institutions. This highlights how the making of "global" issues is not only related to how things travel and keep their shape between "local" and "global", but also within the localities of the "global". Similar to historical past and context, neither "the global" nor "the local" are uniform or stable. Furthermore, as within the relation between text and context, the local is integral to – and not external to – "the global". This also highlights how the global is heterogeneous; the global is multiple. Rather than being a pre-given stable unity external to, and often perceived as standing above, the local, the global can better be seen as a current outcome of an on-going process of *connecting locals*.

# 6. Ordering complexities: On making avian influenza outbreaks governable

*On Saturday February 19, 2008 Şefarettin Yılmaz's hens suddenly became dizzy and exhibited strange behaviour. Earlier that day he had bought 45kg of wheat at the market; he feared that the hens had become ill from the new feed. Their condition quickly worsened, and five out of the twenty hens died. Fearing they were poisoned, he called the village headman who called a veterinarian. Şefarettin Yılmaz and his family kept their 20 hens in the garden of their house in Sazköy, a village by the Black Sea coast. Şefarettin Yılmaz's suspicions that the hens were poisoned were soon forgotten as the fatal disease was defined as* kuş gribi, *or bird flu, caused by the HPAI (H5N1) virus. Before culling and other disease control measures began, 17 birds in the flock had died.*[1]

During a few weeks in the early 2008, what international institutions and national authorities had prepared for, for example with the making of the avian influenza strategies analysed in the previous chapters of this volume, happened: a series of H5N1 HPAI virus outbreaks were detected in the north-western part of Turkey. After the initial outbreak in Sazköy, recalled in the text above, five other outbreaks followed; the outbreak areas were located in relative proximity to the Black Sea. Additionally, one last outbreak was detected close to the Greek border, still close enough in time and space to be defined as part of the same wave of outbreaks. This chapter focuses on these outbreaks. The map that appears in Chapter 2 has also been included below, in order to provide contextualization and to position the location of the outbreak areas and the locations where I have carried out fieldwork relevant to this chapter. The full country map is minimised and the marked areas, covering the so-called 2008 Black Sea outbreak areas, are enlarged. The numbers inserted on this version of the map indicate the sequence in which the outbreaks were reported. As will be discussed, the time of reporting does not necessarily coincide with the date of infection; however, as a matter of simplicity as well as for analytical purposes, I use the numbers to mark these places on this map.

1 Sevindik, Durmuş, Seçkin Kirarslan, Ünal Uzun 2008

2 Date of reporting as reported in Newman, Scott H., Nick Honhold, Javier Sanz-Alvarez and Kiraz Erciyas 2008. The original map is made by U.S. Central Intelligence Agency 2006 but edited by me for the purpose of this project.

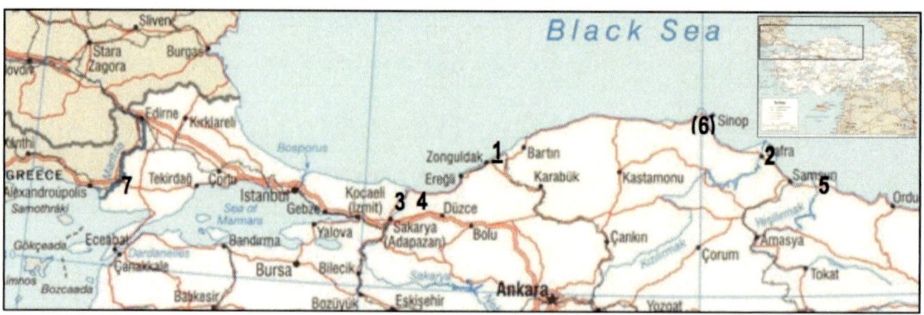


*Name of place and province of HPAI H5N1 outbreaks in February and March 2008 listed according to time of reporting: 1: Sazköy, Zonguldak, 2: Yörükler, Samsun, 3: Yeniçam, Sakarya, 4: Konacık, Sakarya, 5: Aybeder, Samsun, 6: Taşmanlı, Sinop (no field trip to this location), 7: Esetçe, Ipsala/Edirne.[2] Reference of original map: U.S. Central Intelligence Agency 2006. This map is modified by the author based on the outbreak investigation reports referred to in this chapter.*

These outbreaks were investigated by the small but productive group of international experts referred to in this book as the AI project.[3] One of their tasks involved assisting Turkish authorities in epidemiological investigations of these and other outbreaks that took place in the country during the project period. With reference to the epidemiological findings of the two first outbreaks, a special joint mission was initiated and carried out by experts from the FAO and the EU; Turkish experts also assisted with this mission. This joint mission will be discussed in this chapter.

Regarding the AI project, the primary aim of their outbreak investigations was "[t]o investigate the possible source of the Avian Influenza outbreak[s] ( . . . ) and to evaluate the effectiveness of the preventive and control measures".[4] Furthermore, as discussed in the previous two chapters, the outbreak investigation reports were also sent to the FAO, the OIE and the European Union, where they contributed to informing international policy. Hence, these outbreak investigations may be seen as an answer to what the agricultural ecologist Ian Scoones refers to as the "missing middle" between actual outbreak places "on the ground" and the broader policy "at the top".[5]

Through his interdisciplinary research on national and international re-

3 The AI project is the EU funded "Technical Assistance to Avian Influenza Preparedness & Response Project" that was assigned to support the Turkish Government in handling avian influenza in Turkey. Please refer to Chapter 2 of this book for a general overview of this project.

4 Van den Ende, Rinus and Ragip Bayraktar 2008 Sazkoy: 4; Ivanov, Yanko and Ragip Bayraktat 2008 Yorukler 2008: 4

5 Scoones, Ian 2010: 215

sponse to the pandemic avian influenza threat, Scoones pays attention to how, "'high reliability professionals' (...) are currently absent from the international effort – creating a missing middle, a vacuum at the heart of the [disease] response."[6] By calling for "high reliability professionals", he is connecting international disease response to the field of high reliability organizations (HRO), an area researched by Emery Roe and Paul Schulman.[7] Roe and Schulman's "reliability professionals" are the controllers, technical supervisors and department heads of the Californian power grid; they are the "middle-level personnel" possessing the experience, knowledge and ability to make the grid work despite design errors. Roe and Schulman advocate more power to these "middle men" including their right to veto design changes passed down from above. High reliability professionals are valuable in relation to disease response because of their vital positions in critical centres, their knowledge and experience, and as Scoones emphasises, their ability to "track between local understandings of particular situations and unfolding scenarios and the macro situations." Scoones argues that while these professionals play a vital role in operating the high reliability systems of large power grids, they are missing in the international disease response:

> In response to disease emergence these ['high reliability professionals'] would be the people who would make sense of what was happening on the ground, where a disease was first spotted, and the broader policy, liaising between agencies. This vital role is absent because authoritative knowledge, often codified in simple models and plans which do not accept uncertainty, ignorance or complexity, is created only at the top through particular types of expertise. The problem, as the avian influenza story has shown so vividly, is that this is not enough.[8]

In line with Scoones' call for high reliability professionals to make sense of what is happening "on the ground", the Global Strategy points at "weak" epidemiological expertise as one of the major "[c]hallenges and constraints to HPAI control".[9] The Global Strategy establishes national and regional "incorporat[ion of] epidemiological studies linked to disease control programmes to generate quantitative and geo-referenced data on infection and transmission dynamics" as "vital".[10] According to the Global Strategy, the reason for this is

6 Scoones, Ian 2010: 215, regarding 'high reliability professionals' Scoones refers to Roe and Schulman 2008

7 Scoones is referring to Roe and Schulman 2008, but for other classical contributions see also Perrow, Charles 1999; For recent contributions, see Nævestad, Tor-Olav 2009

8 Scoones, Ian 2010: 215

9 FAO, OIE and WHO 2005 Nov: 15, 16

10 *Op. cit.*

that "[s]uch information can provide a *sound basis* for the control and prevention of HPAI."[11] The need for strengthened international support specifically related to epidemiological analysis of disease outbreaks is further stressed in the revised Global Strategy published in 2007, two years after the first Global Strategy was published.[12] Hence, these global strategy documents echo what Scoones and Paul Forster, in their extensive paper on the international avian influenza response, refer to as "the contemporary mantra" of public policy, so-called *evidence-based policy.*[13] Within the public health area, solutions to complex, uncertain and contested matters are sought in normative data, through "sound science" and via "science based approaches", as they, in line with the Global Strategy, are expected to provide a "sound basis for the control and prevention of HPAI".[14]

I will argue that in my study of avian influenza in Turkey the AI project filled the gap identified as the "missing middle" by Scoones, or the lack of epidemiological expertise "linked to disease control programmes" addressed by the Global Strategy. While the personnel, the working conditions and work relations of the AI project team, including their cooperation with local and national collaborators, differ in several ways to the high reliability personnel in Roe and Schulman's study, there are some similarities nonetheless. Using Scoones words, the AI project team, in cooperation with representatives from local and national authorities, were the "people who [made] sense of what was happening on the ground, where a disease was first spotted".[15]

The AI project's epidemiological investigations of outbreak places and the reports thereof that were sent to the FAO, the OIE and the EU continue to provide useful epidemiological information to the international community and represent interesting sites for study avian influenza. Thus, this chapter seeks to study how "sense making on the ground" contributes to enacting avian influenza outbreaks. Drawing on the analytical concepts introduced in previous chapters, this chapter aims to address following questions: how do these outbreak investigations contribute to the *ordering*[16] of avian influenza? How do

[11] FAO, OIE and WHO 2005 Nov: 16, *italics added*

[12] FAO and OIE 2007 March. My reasons for concentrating on the two 2005 editions of the Global Strategy is explained in Chapter 4.

[13] Scoones, Ian and Paul Forester 2008: 64

[14] Scoones, Ian and Paul Forester 2008: 64; see also Stirling, Andy S. and Ian Scoones 2009 with reference to FAO, OIE and WHO 2005 Nov: 16, *italics added.*

[15] Scoones, Ian 2010: 215

[16] E.g. Law, John 1994

the *inscriptions*[17] of these events contribute to *textualizing*[18] the reality of avian influenza, or in other words, how are the outbreak investigations and written reports through which these events are *materialized* and *realized*[19] contributing to *enacting*[20] avian influenza outbreaks? Moreover, I will consider how outbreak investigations involve *contexting*,[21] ordering and enacting matters of bio(*in*)security.[22]

Scoones might be right when he asserts that there are a lack of "people who (...) make sense of what... [is] happening on the ground" when diseases like avian influenza occur. The HPAI outbreaks in Turkey may represent an exception in that they have been the objects of thorough epidemiological investigations. In this chapter, I will utilize the opportunity provided by the reports from these outbreak investigations and by my field studies in Turkey, which coincided with the Sazköy outbreak (as discussed at the beginning of this chapter; the area is marked 1 on the map) to study this matter further. I arrived at Sazköy one week after the outbreak was reported, at which time the village was still being subjected to various biosecurity restrictions, including the controlled movement of humans and vehicles. At this time, the AI project was also carrying out follow-up investigations at the outbreak area and its surroundings. I used the opportunity to interview the village headman and experts from the AI project. I visited six out of the seven 2008 Black Sea outbreak areas; Taşmanlı in Sinop province, marked (6) on the map, was the only area I was unable visit.[23] Hence, methodologically, this chapter juxtaposes various sites, including the outbreak investigation reports, observations from my own

---

17 Latour, Bruno 1999; Latour, Bruno and Steve Woolgar 1979

18 Asdal, Kristin 2008a; 2008b; 2011a; 2014

19 *Ibid.*

20 Mol, Annemarie 2002 See also Asdal, Kristin 2007; 2008c; 2011a.

21 In the previous chapter I discussed the productive coupling of context and Science and Technology Studies (STS) and a performative approach to context*ing*. As mentioned, "context*ing*" as an analytical concept is suggested by Asdal, Kristin and Moser, Ingunn (Eds.) 2012.

22 As discussed in previous chapters, Steve Hinchliffe, John Allen, Stephanie Lavau, Nick Bingham and Simon Carter (2012) suggest a turn away from simple topographic approach towards topology in disease control In Chapter 3 of this book I call attention to bio*in*security as interrelated with, but too often implicit of, what is referred to as biosecurity.

23 For an overview of the field trips, please refer to Chapter 2. The outbreak place I did not visit is located in Sinop Province. Regarding my field trip to Yeniçam village in Sakarya Province, I chose not to make further attempts to reach the outbreak village after meeting difficulties while trying to arrange transportation from this town to the village. This was the only time and place I felt threatened during my field trips. My trip ended few kilometres from the outbreak village I still made observations that, as I in this chapter will show, add to the outbreak investigation reports on the district.

fieldwork and additional resources such as maps, news articles and other kinds of reports, in order to study the ordering of avian influenza outbreaks.

In response to Scoones, I will suggest that the outbreak investigations carried out in these outbreak areas in Turkey can be perceived as filling the "missing middle". Grasping the opportunity provided by occasions where this "missing middle" was filled, this chapter studies how outbreak investigations contribute to ordering the events "on the ground" in ways that make the inscribed versions of the outbreaks mobile and able to inform decisions and policy "at the top"; it will examine how the outbreak investigation team have worked as "reliability professionals" and "middle men" given that their reports are filling this so-called missing middle between the outbreaks "on the ground" and policy making "on the top". Furthermore, this chapter seeks to answer the following: how does filling the "missing middle" contribute to connecting the "ground" with the "top"? Finally, how might a concept of *networking locals* contribute to re-thinking vertical approaches to local – global or transnational relations?

I will explore how the *three tools for ordering* are at work in outbreak investigation reports. Thus, I draw on Kristin Asdal's notion of "tools of democracy", and John Laws notion of "modes of ordering". Asdal acknowledges the way Bruno Latour criticises "political philosophy for having been the victim of a strong object avoidance tendency."[24] Drawing on Latour, Asdal wants to pay attention to "what is at issue, the *res* – the case – that creates a public around it ( . . . ) [O]ne might ask, what is an issue in the first place? How do scientific and technical entities or objects become issues?"[25] By studying outbreaks in this chapter, I aim to come closer to my object, avian influenza, in order to explore how it becomes an issue.

Starting with the *textual inscription of space,* I will explore how outbreak places are being ordered and textually inscribed in the outbreak reports. By studying written reports, field notes and other textual sites, I will also pay attention to how alternative versions of these outbreak places are enacted. Subsequently, I will move onto *maps,* which I, in accordance with Latour, see as another form of inscription, in order to see how they contribute to the ordering of outbreak places. I will engage both with the maps used in the reports and with alternative maps in order to explore alternative versions of these places. The third tool of ordering I will study is what I call *copy/paste tools.* This I will do by following certain pieces of identical text that appear in several

24 Asda, Kristin 2008b: 13, with reference to Latour, Bruno 2005: 16.

25 *Op. cit.*

documents. The words and sentences are the same, but I will pay attention to how they work in the different settings and how they contribute to the ordering and re-ordering of avian influenza by moving from one place to another. The chapter will round off with reflections on how these tools contribute to the epidemiological investigations and reporting and thus to the ordering of avian influenza.

While analysing these tools, I will pay attention to what I characterize as three complementary approaches to heterogeneous objects.[26] Seen as a heterogeneous object, how might the various avian influenza versions co-exist at an outbreak place in ways that are making the different parts "realize capacities for the other"?[27] Moreover, are there ways in which interactions between different versions contribute to *realizing something new*, and/or are there ways in which one version contributes in *disarticulating alternatives*?[28] The latter involves tracing processes, or modes of ordering, through which matters are made present, possibly at the cost of other matters that may be made absent. Hence, ordering is also about inclusion and exclusion, which are of central concern to feminist technoscience scholars who tended to assume a relation between being excluded and being marginalized.[29] One ambition of feminist STS scholars is to foster inclusion as means of empowerment. How might studying avian influenza outbreaks and the reporting thereof – which I will suggest may also be understood as middle-ground processes – contribute to re-thinking the relations between inclusion/exclusion on the one hand and marginalization/empowerment on the other?

## Tool for ordering I: Textual inscription of space

### Field notes 30.01.2008, Sazköy village, Caycuma district, Zonguldak province:

*The minibus stopped by what the driver told me was* Muhtar's çiftlik, *[Muhtar is the village headman and* çiftlik*means farm], at the entrance of the village. (… ) a young man who appeared to be Mohtar's oldest son, came out from the poultry house and met us by the gate. A huge banner was put up at the opposite side of the road from the farm, informing that there was bird flu*

---

26 This is in accordance to discussion in Chapter 2 of this book.

27 Strathern, Marilyn [1991] 2004:39 drawing on Haraway, Donna 1985; Mol, Annemarie 2002.

28 See Asdal, Kristin 2014; Moser Ingunn 2008; Tsing, Anna 2005

29 See Asdal, Kristin, Brita Brenna and Ingunn Moser (Eds.) 2007

*in the village. The son took me by car the approximately 0.5 km to the* kahve *[coffeehouse] in the village centre where Muhtar met me. (…)*

*Inside the* kahve *I was offered tea, and the friendly Muhtar started to talk. (…) [After quite a while, as I was uncertain how he would react when I brought up this topic] I asked Muhtar about his* kumeş *[coop or henhouse], that I had seen when leaving the minibus. The last 8 years or so he grew broilers for* Beypiliç, *he told me. A couple of months ago he started to grow for [another firm] instead. This was the second stock he grew, and it will be "done" at the age of 36 or 37 days (…), because of the bird flu threat [normally broilers are fattened for 42–45 days].*

The broiler farm immediately caught my attention on arrival at Sazköy village, the area where the first of the so-called Black Sea outbreaks in Turkey was detected in January 2008. It was not only its very visible *presence* next to the road at the village entrance that made me so aware of the farm, it caught my attention because of its total *absence* in the preliminary outbreak report that I had read before visiting the village. The outbreak investigation report, written by the AI project, provides extensive and detailed descriptions and illustrations of the area surrounding the "infected house and garden".[30] However, Muhtar's poultry farm does not appear in the report. How does the ordering of outbreak places involve making absence and presence, and how does it affect the reality that is being enacted?[31]

In the following section, I will study how this and the other 2008 Black Sea outbreaks were textually inscribed through outbreak investigation reports. Juxtaposing sites also enables me to see how these inscriptions involve exclusions as well as inclusions, hence how a "lack of links, of relations, may also shape" avian influenza "in certain ways".[32] How do outbreak investigations involve textual making of absence and presence and in which ways does this contribute to making avian influenza matter? Moreover, how does it contribute to disarticulating alternatives?[33]

Asdal illustrates how "issues are shaped not only through the knitting of alliances and relations but also through exclusions, through arguments and relations that are cut off or never allowed to circulate or move beyond their local

[30] Van den Ende, Rinus and Ragip Bayraktar 2008 Sazkoy: 6

[31] Ingunn Moser's notions of absence and presence was introduced in Chapter 1 and used in Chapter 3 of this volume

[32] Asdal, Kristin 2007: 318

[33] Moser, Ingunn 2008

site in the first place."[34] In regards to Muhtar's coop, the epidemiologist later explained that there was no need to include the farm in the report as the poultry house had been checked and no sign of disease among the broilers were detected.[35] Does it matter that this poultry house does not appear in the outbreak report despite the fact that it was positioned well within the so-called 3-kilometre protection zone around the centre of the outbreak? How do the exclusions and inclusions influence the way the topology of outbreak places – or sites of bio*in*security – are being textually inscribed?

## Enacting space: Inscribing natural features and non-human actors

The outbreak investigation reports describe outbreak places in a precise and detailed way:

> Location: Sazköy village (41034'03,00"N 32004'15,65"E) is situated along the Filyos river, a branch of which is forming a coastal lagoon(…). This lagoon apparently is an attractive resting/feeding station to aquatic birds on their migration over or along the Black Sea.[36]

Starting with practical information on the mission team, dates of visit and so on, the outbreak investigation report on the Sazköy outbreak is, in this text, turning towards the outbreak place, where it is letting the location unfold: a riverside, a "resting/feeding station" for migrating aquatic birds, is inscribed. The report provides detailed and picturesque illustrations, sharing the wonderful "view from the lagoon" with the reader through four sunny pictures included in the appendix of the report. In this way, the outbreak investigation report is assembling, ordering and inscribing features, which contribute to enacting the location; it is textualizing a particular version of reality, hence it is enacting a particular topology of the outbreak place.

The second outbreak that was reported and investigated, in Yörükler village, Samsun province, appears to be of a very similar character to the first one:

> Location: Samsun province lies on the Black Sea coast of Turkey, 400 km northeast of Ankara. The province contains two large wetland areas, one (the delta of the Kizilirmak River) in Bafra district and the other (the delta of the Yesilirmak River) in Carsamba district.

---

[34] Asdal, Kristin 2007: 318

[35] Personal communication with an epidemiological expert in Ankara 29.01.2008

[36] Van den Ende, Rinus and Ragip Bayraktar 2008 Sazkoy: 4

[two country maps are here pointing out the location of the outbreak, alone and in relation to the previous outbreak in Sazöy]

These are the deltas of two of the largest rivers in Turkey. Large numbers of migratory waterfowl pass through these areas in spring and autumn. The Kizilirmak Delta, a natural site with an undisturbed flora and fauna, covers an area of 70.000 hectares. 350 bird species were discovered in this area where around 100,000 migrant and non-migrant birds spend the winter(…)

Domestic poultry (… ) are found close to these wetland areas which flood seasonally, leading to closer proximity between wild and domestic birds at times of the year when wildfowl numbers are highest.[37]

In this report, the detailed descriptions *include* specific features: wetlands, rivers and migratory waterfowl. The site is further enacted as "natural", "undisturbed" and "large"; it has "large wetland areas", "two of the largest rivers in Turkey", and the "numbers of migratory waterfowl" are "[l]arge". Hence, the report produces a particular image, not only of the immediate surroundings of the specific outbreak place, but of the whole province. The whole Samsun province is enacted as "two large wetland areas", dominated by a remarkably high abundance of migratory and non-migratory wild birds. Much like the report on the first outbreak, this description enacts the outbreak place and the wider surroundings as a wild bird habitat; 12 pictures are included which show "[v]iews from lagoon".[38]

In addition to wild birds, the report on this second reported outbreak is also including and making present "1.5 million backyard poultry", further contributing to the representation of Samsun province.[39] In this way, the first step in ordering the outbreak place is about *inclusions*; inclusions of "large", "undisturbed", "natural" "wetlands", and of a large population of wild (migratory) birds and backyard poultry.

This relatively homogeneous kind of place is also a result of exclusions and the making of absence. For example, when the report makes it clear that "[t]here is no commercial poultry establishments *in the wetland area*", the outbreak investigation report is ensuring the absence of commercial poultry.[40] Moreover, the report is drawing in outbreaks that were confirmed to have occurred in different places in the province in 2006. By conveying that "[n]one [of the outbreaks] were in commercial sector birds", the report is excluding the

[37] Ivanov, Yanko and Ragip Bayraktar 2008 Yorukler: 4–6

[38] Ivanov, Yanko and Ragip Bayraktar 2008 Yorukler: Annex2 pp. 17–22

[39] Ivanov, Yanko and Ragip Bayraktar 2008 Yorukler: 6

[40] Ivanov, Yanko and Ragip Bayraktar 2008 Yorukler: 12, *emphasis added*

commercial poultry sector, making the sector absent from the outbreak place, "the wetlands" and from the Samsun province as a whole.[41]

Based on my field trips to Sazköy and the impression I got from travelling around in Samsun a few months before the outbreak, it is clear that these places could have been enacted differently; both the province in general and areas close to Yörükler village in particular offer other features that may contribute in enacting different versions of these places. For example, when travelling through the town close to Yörükler, Bafra, I noticed widespread activity related to commercial poultry production. During that field trip, I mainly talked with ornithologists, as I was undertaking a wild bird catching technique course organized by the AI project.[42] Similar to the epidemiologists carrying out the investigations of the Yörükler outbreak, my attention was directed towards the wetlands rather than towards the surrounding farmlands, the backyard poultry or the network of commercial poultry production. A poultry meat report for Samsun province, published by the district agricultural authorities, *İl Tarım Müdürlüğü,* thus provides a useful supplement to my limited impressions of the sector.[43]

The image of Samsun province enacted in the poultry meat report is very different to that in the outbreak investigation report. The poultry meat report is textualizing Samsun as a place with strong ambitions to develop the commercial poultry sector. The poultry meat report illustrates how two main commercial producers were already playing an important role in the province. These producers had contracting farms in most districts around the province at the time of the outbreak. The poultry meat report is bringing in a different version of Samsun province than the version enacted by the outbreak investigation report, and supports what I saw during my field trip, namely widespread activity related to commercial poultry production.

### Varying criteria for getting access and being inscribed

How is it possible that the commercial poultry sector has not been included in these reports? As the experience of Muhtar's poultry house in Sazköy demon-

41 Ivanov, Yanko and Ragip Bayraktar 2008 Yorukler: 6. Commercial poultry is mentioned only one more time in the report, then in relation to surveillance and with reference to an Avian influenza manual rather than to Samsun as a place for commercial poultry production: "Active surveillance and monitoring should be carried out of wild birds, backyard and commercial poultry according to Avian influenza surveillance manual" (p. 15).

42 Please refer to Chapter 2 for an overview of my field trips. The mentioned Wild Bird Caching Technique Course took place in the districts Atakum and Yörükler of Samsun Province and we drove through Bafra district on the way between these two course sites.

43 Altındeğer, Mustafa and Burhan Hekimoğlu 2010

strates, absence of both clinical signs and positive laboratory tests work as means justifying that the commercial sector is not included; that they are not inscribed and reported. Hence, due to lack of evidence of infection, commercial poultry do not contribute to enacting outbreak places. This criterion for inclusion does not apply to wild birds and sites that may be associated with these birds.

In relation to the Sazköy outbreak, no wild birds tested positive for H5N1. However, a dead swan found by the AI project team in a lagoon well within the 3-kilometre protection zone contributed to establishing a lagoon outbreak – or a wildlife outbreak. The report is creating expectations of this bird and its' fellow species members:

> An interesting point is the remark by hunters that there is a tradition of never killing swans. This explains the presence of a group of very tame juvenile Mute Swans which now act as sentinel birds for virus presence in the lagoon. (It is expected that H5N1 will be retrieved from the swan carcass submitted to the Etlik VCR on the 22$^{nd}$January.)[44]

According to the same outbreak investigation report, the initial results of the tests carried out by the national reference laboratory at Etlik were negative. However, the report states that an "[e]gg inoculation was carried out and results are pending."[45] Hence, the option remains open that the swan may have carried the virus. The final results of the egg inoculation were not available at the time when the report was written, thus the "lagoon outbreak" remains, and the clearest evidence persists – despite no findings of virus in wild birds, not even in the swans pointed out here as sentinel birds. Moreover, when the egg inoculation test failed to produce positive results a few days, the "Sazkoy lagoon outbreak" was not withdrawn.[46] While the lagoon outbreak remained, it is not mentioned in further reports. However, the swans and the geographical features that were inscribed and contributed to textually enacting this outbreak place, had already laid the ground for a focus on wildlife. During the following weeks, only one wild bird would come to test positive for H5N1 infection.

---

44 Van den Ende, Rinus and Bayraktar, Ragip 2008 Sazkoy: 10

45 *Op. cit.*

46 Two mute swan carcasses were found during the outbreak investigation, but initially only one was tested (the swan that appeared in the text above). As no positive results were retrieved from this carcass, the other carcass was collected by the AI project team when they carried out a follow-up visit to the village together with representatives from national and local authorities on 31.01.2008. The epidemiologists were hoping this carcass would provide proof for wildlife involvement. However, according to one of the epidemiologists, the results were negative.

That was a moribund buzzard which was found at the Yörükler outbreak area and whose role in infect*ing* or as infect*ed by* local poultry remains unknown.[47]

While wild birds were included simply because of their presence, commercial poultry required positive results on laboratory tests in order to be included in the reports. As the latter never transpired, the outbreak reports could produce and re-produce a specific topography – free from elements associated with commercial poultry. The different inclusion criteria for wild and domestic birds contributes to a separation, where wild birds and what is associated with these are inscribed and made mobile, while other matters remain and are not made mobile; hence they are not make to matter.

What we have seen so far is how the outbreak investigation reports concerning the outbreaks in Sazköy and Yörükler are inscribing particular spatial features; i.e., how they are textualizing a certain topology of bio*in*security: Both places are enacted as wetland areas and attractive wild bird habitats where wild birds and backyard poultry live close together. At the same time, juxtaposing the outbreak investigation reports with field notes, observations and alternative reports contribute to enacting alternative versions of the areas, which make us aware of the absence of commercial poultry production in these documents.[48] The possible presence of any commercial poultry production only appears indirectly and with assurances that the sector is not involved. In this way, exclusion and inclusion, but also lack of inclusion, contribute to the ordering of outbreak places where wild birds and backyard poultry are present and act together, while commercial poultry is absent. Thus, the scene is set for a possible version of events. But, who else is involved in enacting this scene and what role do they play?

47 Newman, Scott H., Nick Honhold, Javier Sanz-Alvarez and Kiraz Erciyas 2008. This bird will re-appear in the next, concluding chapter of this volume

48 Another example on how activities related to commercial poultry production have been excluded from outbreak sites can be found in the twopage version of the report on the Sazköy outbreak prepared by the Ministry of Agriculture and Rural Affairs. The front page of this report explicitly states: "No laying hen holding exists within the surveillance zone"(MARA/KKGM 2008 Sazkoy: 1, *underlined in original as only sentence on the page*) The inattentive reader may assume that this means no commercial poultry production takes place within the 3-kilomtre protection zone, however the report only discusses the nonexistence of any *laying hen holding* in the area; it does not make any claims about broiler farms within the 3-kilomtre protection zone.

## Inscribing human actors and cultural activities

Sazköy and Yörukler are both characterized as villages "with a lively hunting tradition".[49] In both reports, the general introduction of the outbreak place is followed by a section on hunting. This is the only place where we get a glimpse of the people living in these villages. Thus, hunters are the only human actors that are textualized in the reports. Interviews with hunters establish the importance of hunting for the majority of households at these specific places: 60% of the households are said to "have members who are actively hunting".[50] Furthermore, the interviews reveal that hunters sometimes find ringed birds which they, according to the reports, "promised to save ( . . . ) in order to help tracing of migrant waterfowl."[51] In this way, hunters are given a role in disease surveillance.

Moreover, hunters are given a direct role in the introduction of the disease. In the outbreak investigation report pertaining to Sazköy, a family member of the infected household "volunteered the information of having shot 3 Mallard and 4 Woodcocks" three days before the backyard poultry turned ill.[52] The hunted birds were reportedly "cleaned for consumption on that same day in the backyard. The scraps were unceremoniously disposed [of] in the garden [where the infected backyard poultry was kept]."[53] Thus, this hunter and his family members are given the role in the conclusion of the Sazköy outbreak investigation report, as the bridge for the virus, connecting the wild birds (hunted birds) with the domestic birds (scavenging backyard poultry). As no remains were left of these birds, it was not possible to test the birds to ascertain whether they were carriers of the virus. Still, they are acting as *the* only possible source of infection in the report.[54]

---

49 Van den Ende, Rinus and Ragip Bayraktar 2008 Sazkoy: 6, and Ivanov, Yanko and Ragip Bayraktar 2008 Yörükler: 8

50 Van den Ende, Rinus and Ragip Bayraktar 2008 Sazkoy: 9; Ivanov, Yanko and Ragip Bayraktar 2008 Yörükler: 12, in the case of Yörükler it is stated that " (60%) have members who are actively hunting and fishing." It thus remains uncertain how many who are actually actively hunting as the number also refers to fishing. For the sake of my argument, the number (60%) contributes to establish hunting as a widespread activity in the report.

51 Ivanov, Yanko and Ragip Bayraktar 2008 Yorukler: 12. For an almost identical sentence see Van den Ende, Rinus and Ragip Bayraktar 2008 Sazkoy: 9.

52 Van den Ende, Rinus and Ragip Bayraktar 2008 Sazkoy: 9

53 *Op. cit.*

54 This theory for introduction is further emphasized in the FAO-EU Joint Mission report which suggests hunted birds were a source of infection in four of the six outbreak areas (Newman, Scott H., and Nick Honhold, Javier Sanz-Alvarez, Kiraz Erciyas 2008).

Following up on the reflections from the section above, it ought to be noted that poultry owners remain invisible, silent and not included in the outbreak investigation report. Thus, the report does not mention that the owner of the infected poultry in Sazköy had recently brought new feed from the market – this was only mentioned in newspaper reports, one of which was referenced in the introduction of this chapter. I was told that feed was not relevant for the report due to the incubation period, as the time between the birds being fed the new feed and the onset of clinical signs was too short,[55] hence there was no need to include this in the report. Neither was any other food sources included, except the mentioned "unceremoniously disposed" remains of wild birds brought to the household by a hunter.[56]

Consequently, hunters possess the *only* human role that may directly have contributed to introduction of the disease. While a relation between hunting and the introduction of disease has been made in Sazköy, this was not possible in Yörükler.[57] However, despite the lack of such a link in Yörükler, this is compensated for by the above-mentioned ways of establishing hunting as more common than not among the households in this area in general. Additionally, hunting is made significant for this latter outbreak, for example by stating that the outbreak investigation team observed "[s]everal hunters", and by claiming that "[m]any villagers however continue to indulge in some degree of opportunistic hunting outside the official seasons." In the case of Yörükler, the outbreak investigation report conveys a lack of certainty as to whether hunting was the reason for the introduction of disease, or if the introduction was caused by direct contact between wild and domestic birds. The latter possibility was enabled by the way natural features of the outbreak site were ordered and textualized: as a wetland area, a densely populated wild bird habitat, and a place where wild birds and scavenging backyard poultry lived side by side.

So far, studying the textual inscription of space shows how complex outbreak situations are being ordered through outbreak investigations and in the

---

55 Personal communication with epidemiological expert Ankara 31.01.2008

56 Van den Ende, Rinus and Ragip Bayraktar 2008 Sazkoy

57 The initial outbreak investigation report on this outbreak, on which I have so far build my analysis (Ivanov, Yanko and Ragip Bayraktar 2008 Yorukler), does just not mention whether members of the household were involved in hunting or if hunted birds were brought to the house. In a later outbreak investigation report (Newman, Scott H. and Nick Honhold, Javier Sanz-Alvarez, Kiraz Erciyas 2008) it is however explicitly stated that members of the infected household in Yorukler "stated No( . . . )" to the investigator's question regarding hunting. In this report, we can see that members of this household denied that their poultry had been in "[d]irect contact with remains of hunted birds", however, this latter report refuses to accept this and conveys: "[s]tated "No" but possible".

reporting thereof. By textually inscribing outbreak places, these documents are ordering space and enacting a certain kind of place. As Latour argues, inscriptions are also making things, in this case outbreak places, mobile; they are immutable mobiles, allowing readers to gain an impression of the sites from a distance. Hence, the sites that readers see from a distance, or the kinds of places these reports are enacting, consist of what is included in the reports, the matters that are made present: wetlands, densely co-inhabited by high numbers of wild birds, backyard poultry and hunters. Materialized in the form of outbreak reports, these outbreak places may travel internationally and, as we saw already in the previous two chapters, contribute to policy-making and the development of strategies.[58]

What is excluded, or simply not included, is left behind and are not made mobile. Still they may have effect on the version that travel; the absence of alternatives that do not become mobile may strengthen the versions that do travel.[59] Hence, according to the outbreak investigation reports – the version that reaches the international community – these two first reported outbreaks, which would soon became part of a "wave" of seven outbreaks, "might well serve to illustrate the *fact* that H5N1 can be introduced in Turkey by migratory birds."[60] Consequently, the next matter of concern is then, how does this "fact" produced through the investigations of the two first 2008 Black Sea outbreaks have effect?

## Local outbreak places become centres of international attention

The conclusions from the investigations of these two outbreaks caught the attention of FAO's Chief of Animal Health Service, Joseph Domenech. On February 4, 2008 Domenech sent an official request to the Chief Veterinary Officer of the Turkish Ministry of Agriculture, Dr. Haluk Aşkaroğlu. Domenech asked permission to send a team to Turkey in order to investigate the role of wild birds in relation to H5N1 HPAI.[61] The Turkish authorities responded positively. Aşkaroğlu ensured the ministry's full collaboration and also stated that

58 In chapters 4 and 5 I argued that inscriptions might be immutable mobiles in line with Latour's argument, but that they may also change on the way. This calls for attention to how they may as well be mutable mobiles. I will return to this point later in the current chapter.

59 Asdal, Kristin 2007

60 Van den Ende, Rinus and Ragip Bayraktar 2008 Sazkoy: 11; Ivanov, Yanko and Ragip Bayraktar 2008 Yörükler: 13, *emphasis added*

61 Newman, Scott H., Nick Honhold, Javier Sanz-Alvarez and Kiraz Erciyas 2008: Annex1, p. 21

the AI project would partake in this mission.[62] The initial objective of this joint mission was to carry out ornithological studies in relation to the epidemiology of the outbreaks of HPAI in Sazköy and Yörukler.[63]

Four new outbreaks were detected during the weeks the mission was carried out; the joint mission team also investigated these subsequent outbreaks. The four outbreaks taking place during the time of the mission were inscribed in the joint mission report, where also the individual reports on the first two outbreaks, in Sazköy and Yörükler, were re-inscribed. The joint mission did not carry out outbreak investigations of these two first outbreaks, but the outbreak investigation reports on these outbreaks inform the joint mission and are brought along in the joint mission report. The final outbreak, taking place after the joint mission concluded, was inscribed and textualized by the AI project team in an individual report of same format as the Sazköy and Yörükler outbreaks. The parts of the joint mission report which inscribe the findings and results of the outbreak investigations represents a strategic place for my study of "the missing middle" of the investigations of these four outbreaks.[64] In the following section, I will study how the outbreak investigations carried out by this joint mission team contributed in to the ordering of avian influenza. I will keep my attention on the textual inscription of space.

## Re-enacting space

Instead of detailed and picturesque descriptions, the joint mission outbreak investigation uses "spatial analysis" based on numbers and specific questions aimed at identifying possible spatial relations that can shed light on the source of infection and possible ways of spread. A table contributes in the ordering of these spatial relations between detected outbreaks and a range of possible sources of infection. I will study the question addressed in this table that sought to identify "Poultry farms within 3 km".[65] The possible answers, "Yes"

62 Newman, Scott H., Nick Honhold, Javier Sanz-Alvarez and Kiraz Erciyas 2008: Annex1, p. 22

63 Newman, Scott H., Nick Honhold, Javier Sanz-Alvarez and Kiraz Erciyas 2008: 10

64 The results of the outbreak investigations are also presented in Annex 4 of the FAO-EU joint mission report. The ornithological field studies are mentioned in the body text and will be studied further in the following chapter

65 Even though it is not specified whether this is a 3 kilometre straight air line or a 3 kilometre road, it is reasonable to assume it is the former, as this coincides with what is known as the 3-kilometre "protection zone" around the area of outbreak. A "surveillance zone" stretches a further 7 kilometres from this area. Outbreak reports commonly contain a simple map of the outbreak place and surrounding villages where the protection and surveillance zones are highlighted.

or "No", are working to include or exclude poultry farms from the so-called protection zone of 3 km radius of the centre of outbreak. In other words, this question represents an epidemiological tool, or an "inscription device", which is including commercial poultry production to, or excluding it from, the outbreak place. In other words, the table and the variables, "Yes" or "No", contribute to textualizing poultry production as absent or present.[66]

When the AI project's report contributes to fill the cells and re-inscribes the Sazköy outbreak in the joint mission report, Muhtar's coop remains absent. As the coop is not included in the AI project's report, the answer to the question above was 'No' and the table is excluding the possibility of such a source of infection. Also for Yörükler the answer was "No".

After the third reported outbreak investigated and reported by the joint mission, which took place in Konacık village in Sakarya province, the joint mission outbreak investigation report claims that "No" poultry farms exist within a 3 kilometre distance of the centre of the outbreak. Here I had a similar experience as when I arrived Sazköy, though. The farm I introduced when opening Chapter 2, where the helpful minibus driver let me off inside poultry farmers' garden, was only 1200 metres from the outbreak place. On arrival, a young man at the farm told me that the two poultry houses right behind us, which he ran together with his parents, each had the capacity to accommodate 20 000 chickens; moreover, he mentioned they had produced broilers for a company called Şenpiliç for 12–13 years.[67] The young man and his mother assured me that their poultry had not been infected during the outbreak; also, their poultry remained unaffected when the virus killed and the authorities culled the backyard poultry in the neighbourhood. Moreover, this family, and the production system they were part of, were not included when the events were textualized in the joint mission report; a "No" in the table ordering spatial relations in this report clearly excludes this and other "[p]oultry farms within 3 km" from the outbreak place.

At*one* of the six outbreak places, in Yenicam village in Sakarya province, a "Yes" is including "[p]oultry farms within 3 km".[68] Another inscription device did however contribute to neutralizing this farm, as the report makes it clear that "the poultry farm in question was tested and found to be negative both clinically and on sampling. The pattern of disease and the results of testing

[66] Bruno Latour and Steve Woolgar introduced the term "inscription device"' in their book, Laboratory Life (1979); the authors make reference to laboratory equipment (or devices) that work to transform substances into diagrams or figures (inscriptions).

[67] Field notes: Konacık village Karasu District, Sakarya Province, 21.10.2008

[68] Newman, Scott, Honhold, Javier Sanz-Alvarez and Kiraz Erciyas 2008: Annex 4, p. 38.

indicate that this is a very unlikely source of the outbreak."[69] On the one hand, the table includes the farm as part of the outbreak place, and on the other hand, clinical investigations and sampling work together to exclude it, or remove it from the influenza issue at hand.

During my trip to Sakarya province, eight months after these outbreaks, I realized that for the province in general, and even more so for the two districts reporting outbreaks during the time of these Black Sea outbreaks, poultry production was of great importance.[70] Considerable road construction was taking place and I soon gave up trying to remember where I saw large poultry houses from the minibus window. In fact, it would have been impossible for me to visit each one. Both in the Karasu district, where the Konacık outbreak took place, and in Kaynarça district, where one poultry farm was reported to be located within 3 kilometres from the so-called Yenicam outbreak place, I noticed the prevalence of long, low and narrow buildings; most of the buildings had one or two silos attached to one of the short ends. Many coops were shiny and looked new. My field notes from the trip to Yenicam read: "There are many big, and some incredibly big, poultry houses! One of those close to Yenicam is especially big; it has 4 silos!"[71] Travelling through this area with my avian influenza research glasses struck me how it is dominated by on-going and extensive agro-industrial development, or what the global strategy refers to as the "livestock revolution".[72] The official website for Kaynarça district, where Yenicam is located, highlights the significance of the poultry industry in this area. The website states that 650 poultry houses are involved in the expanding commercial poultry sector in the district. Given this large number, it is surprising that the industry is virtually absent in the outbreak investigation reports.[73] The contrast between how this area is enacted in outbreak investigation reports with what I witnessed during my travels, made me realize how outbreak investigations are about reducing complexity. Moreover, the contrast, interference, or "friction" between these versions also made it apparent how

69 Newman, Scott, Honhold, Javier Sanz-Alvarez and Kiraz Erciyas 2008

70 This field trip took place in October 2008, eight months after the last reported outbreak in the province.

71 Field notes 24.10.2008, Kaynarca, Sakarya

72 FAO, OIE and WHO 2005 May; FAO, OIE and WHO 2005 Nov. For a discussion on avian influenza and the "livestock revolution" in the Global Strategy, please refer to Chapter 4.

73 http://www.kaynarca.gov.tr/, accessed on 20.04.2009. Also in the nearby district of Kandira, Turkey production boomed in the early 2000s, however, in 2011 the poultry houses closed "one by one" http://www.aktifhaber.com/kandirada-hindi-ciftlikleri-bir-bir-kapandi-534963h.htm *last read 04.08.2014*. It is unclear what caused this change; also, this issue is beyond the scope of this project.

the ways outbreaks were being ordered and inscribed in the reports involves separation; it made me aware of how inscription of certain matters of concern is also contributing to creating, or *making*, distance to the matters that are not being inscribed, and which in that way are being left behind.[74]

The tools for textual inscription of space differ in the joint mission outbreak investigation report compared to the detailed and picturesque descriptions at work in the AI project's reports on the initial two outbreaks. Nonetheless, the *places* that are being produced are very similar. Both the AI project's reports and the joint mission report are ordering outbreak places in a way that are making backyard poultry and wild birds the main actors, while hardly any room is given to commercial poultry. Examining how the question of "Poultry farms within 3 km" has contributed to the ordering of outbreak places has provided space to study how exclusions are at work when complex outbreak places are ordered into transparent and manageable sites of epidemiological analysis. Studying their so-called "tempo-spatial analysis" will provide a further opportunity to examine how particular features are being included in the joint mission outbreak investigation report.

## Tempo-spatial ordering of objects of investigation

As part of their epidemiological analysis, the joint mission aimed at determining a "pattern of disease" and identifying possible relations between the outbreaks.[75] In order to accomplish this, they performed a "tempo-spatial analysis". These analyses transform spatiality into selected quantitative relations: "Distance of outbreak from coast (km)", "Distance between outbreaks (km)" and "Distance of outbreak from waterbody (km)". In this way, the six outbreaks that were detected before the mission ended were ordered in relation to the Black Sea shore, or alternatively to "significant waterbodies", and in relation to other outbreaks in Turkey reported within this period. Furthermore, the analyses include various dates, such as the date of onset of clinical signs and the date of reporting. In this way the outbreaks are ordered; the complex outbreak places are being turned into well-defined, quantified, lucid entities that enable "basic geometric calculations". In other words, the outbreaks are made governable.[76]

[74] I am drawing on my discussion from Chapter 2 about how Asdal's use of the term "interference" and Tsing's concept of "friction" may contribute to something new.

[75] Newman, Scott H. and Nick Honhold, Javier Sanz-Alvarez, Kiraz Erciyas 2008: Annex 4: p. 33

[76] Newman, Scott H. Nick Honhold, Javier Sanz-Alvarez and Kiraz Erciyas 2008: 7

These analyses and calculations rely on the basic assumption that all outbreaks are detected and reported; that all outbreaks are included and participate in the tempo-spatial overview.[77] The report points at the frequency of samples "submitted from suspect cases for lab testing in the periods between outbreaks". Hence, frequency of samples works, for the joint mission team and in their report, as a reliable indication of efficient reporting, and a reason to assume that the topography of outbreak places represents a coherent and transparent whole.

However, when turning away from general surveillance records and looking at the specificities of individual outbreaks, reporting practices appear to be rather random, coincidental or even absent.[78] Many, if not most, of the reported outbreaks were detected due to coincidence rather than public awareness and well functioning surveillance routines. Drawing in contexts enacted previously in this book enables this argument:[79] As we saw in Chapter 3 and in the introduction of this chapter, the owners of infected poultry (turkeys) in Manyas (2005) and in Sazköy (2008) thought the birds were poisoned, and therefore contacted the village headmen and veterinary authorities. While this has been mentioned in newspaper articles, it is not apparent in the surveillance records. Furthermore, a veterinarian involved in the culling during the countrywide outbreaks in 2006, told me that backyard poultry owners normally do not contact veterinarians when their birds are ill. Rather, the common practice is to slaughter poultry when they show signs of disease and then consume them.[80] This is evident in news reports covering the 2008 outbreak in Yenicam. In one report, a local woman explains that people in her village had slaughtered and eaten ill and dying poultry one month before the outbreak was detected.[81] Lack of reporting when poultry become ill is also raised as a concern in relation to avian influenza surveillance in Turkey by others, the AI project included. In relation to previous outbreaks in Turkey, low awareness and "a lack of early farmer reporting" are obstacles for the detection of the disease, according to the AI project.[82]

77 Newman, Scott H., Nick Honhold, Javier Sanz-Alvarez and Kiraz Erciyas 2008: Annex 4: 32.

78 Also John Law and Ingunn Moser (2011) point at how the epidemiological models they study depend on or include uncertain data contexts.

79 Again I am drawing on Asdal (2012); this time as a tool for self-reflection

80 Personal communication with veterinarian working for the Ağrı provincial veterinary service on 16.06.07. See also AI project 2007; Durutan, Nedret and Okan, Cüneyt 2006; Geerlings, Ellen 2006,

81 Tokuş, Zaferm Arife Balta, Aziz Güvner 2008

82 See Honhold, Nick and Ragip Bayraktar 2007 Diyarbakir and Batman. The outbreak in

These examples show that rather than a coherent topography, it seems reasonable to assume that the outbreaks that are detected and reported, and hence included in the spatial temporal analysis, are more random than coherent. Operating as if the topography of outbreaks were coherent, the joint mission outbreak investigation report does enable the following conclusion of the tempo-spatial analysis:

> This epidemic has the characteristics of a series of separate introductions clustered in time but not space. There is a heavy bias towards the coastline and perhaps towards nearby waterbodies.
>
> There is no indication of a propagating epidemic, which would be expected if poultry to poultry spread were occurring.[83]

The tempo-spatial analysis together with the textualization of outbreak places contributed to establishing coastline and waterbodies as the only relevant spaces for the joint mission to search for the source of introduction. These analyses fit well with the exclusion of poultry as implicated in spread, given "[t]hat there is no indication of a propagating epidemic".[84] The spatial relations of these outbreaks of avian influenza is perhaps most powerful when they are enacted by maps. In the following section, I will move on to study how maps contribute to the ordering and enacting of outbreak places.

## Tools for ordering II: Mapping avian influenza

Maps and text assist each other in showing the position of the individual outbreaks and relations between the centre of the outbreak and other factors considered relevant by the outbreak investigation team, and a variety of maps are used in the outbreak reports. As more outbreaks were detected during the weeks following the one first reported from Sazköy, these other outbreaks also appear on the maps. This section will analyse how maps contribute both to the ordering of individual outbreak places, and how they contribute in enacting connection to possible source of introduction as well as relations between outbreaks.

---

Esetce, reported after the FAO-EU joint mission ended, may contribute in enacting a context from the future that sustains my current argument. According to the AI project's outbreak report this outbreak was identified by coincident by veterinarians who visited the area as part of a rabies vaccination campaign (Van den Ende, Marinus and Ragip Bayraktar 2008 Esetce).

83 Newman, Scott H. Nick Honhold, Javier Sanz-Alvarez and Kiraz Erciyas 2008: Appendix 4: 34

84 *Op. cit.*

## Placing outbreaks on a Turkey map

With their very simple design, indicating national and provincial borders and separating sea and land, the various country maps used in these reports appear to be as neutral as a country map can be. When I choose a map, among the many available on internet, for displaying where in Turkey I have done fieldwork, I also searched for a "neutral map", a map without disturbing details but still enough information to contextualize, to make a connection between this text and "the ground" where I have carried out fieldwork. Simple and neutral as it might appear, the map I chose is indeed named Political Map Turkey 2006. Both the country maps used in the outbreak investigation report and the map I use to display sites for fieldwork, along with the Google maps used in the outbreak investigation reports are powerfully inscribing certain relations and hence contribute to enacting a certain version of avian influenza.

**Figure 1: Location of HPAI outbreaks in Turkey Jan-Feb 2008**

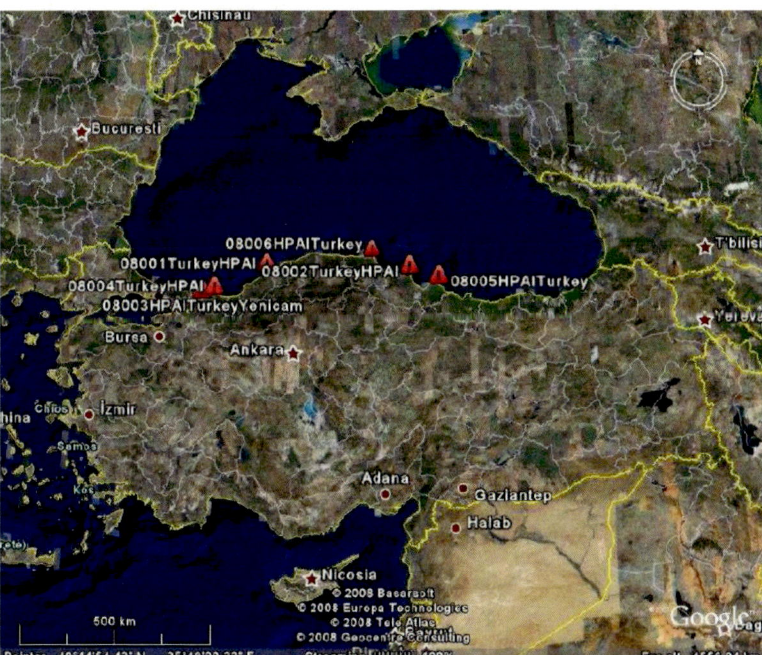


*Google Earth image by © 2008 Basarsoft, © 2008 Europa Technologies, © 2008 Tele Atlas and © 2008 Geocentre Consulting in Newman, Scott H. and Nick Honhold, Javier Sanz-Alvarez, Kiraz Erciyas 2008: 12, and Appendix 4*

The map above is taken from the joint mission report where it appears both in the body text and in the attached outbreak investigation report.[85] This Google map works well to illustrate *where* the outbreaks took place; primarily *where* in the country and *where* in relation to the other outbreaks during these specific weeks, but also *where* in relation to other geographical features. In other words, it contributes to inscribing outbreaks in a particular way and ordering the outbreaks in relation to a specific context. On this map, it is the southern shore of the Black Sea coast that is most visible. Thus, the map, along with the spatial analysis performed by the joint mission, works to establish and re-establish the relation between the individual outbreaks, and between these and the Black Sea coastline.

This map offers an overview over all the outbreaks in this "wave", except the last incident, which was reported after the joint mission ended. With Law, I suggest that this is a way of "looking up"; it is a way to "[s]ee things as a whole" and to "[b]ring in and incorporate elements that were previously separate."[86] Hence, the map may be seen as a way to "understand the complex whole."[87] This is echoing the distinction Strathern makes between a whole image versus an image of a whole. Much like Strathern, Law rejects the possibility of assembling an image of *the* complex whole. Rather, he suggests we should be "looking down" so that "we are discovering complexity in [the] detail"; the map is a whole image, but not an image of a whole.[88] In order to "look down" to attend to specificities, I will also study the individual mapping of the two outbreaks that were first investigated and mapped by the AI project, later to be re-inscribed into the joint mission map, where they contribute, together with the inscription of the following outbreaks, to enacting this wave of outbreaks.

## Looking down at local features

In the Sazköy, Yörükler and Esetçe reports, the specific outbreaks are inscribed on local maps. These are mainly Google maps, where pins are added displaying local features considered relevant by the epidemiologists. I see these maps as tools for inscribing and enacting the context where this particular outbreak

[85] Newman, Scott H. and Nick Honhold, Javier Sanz-Alvarez, Kiraz Erciyas 2008: 12 and Appendix 4. Illustration text too is copied from the mentioned report.

[86] Law, John 2004:16

[87] *Op. cit.*

[88] *Op. cit.*, see also Mol, Annemarie (2002) regarding complex and multiple issues. Strathern, Marilyn 1994

took place.[89] Sazköy appears blurry on this low-resolution Google map taken from the outbreak investigation report and inserted below.[90] As the map covers a relatively large area, few details are visible.

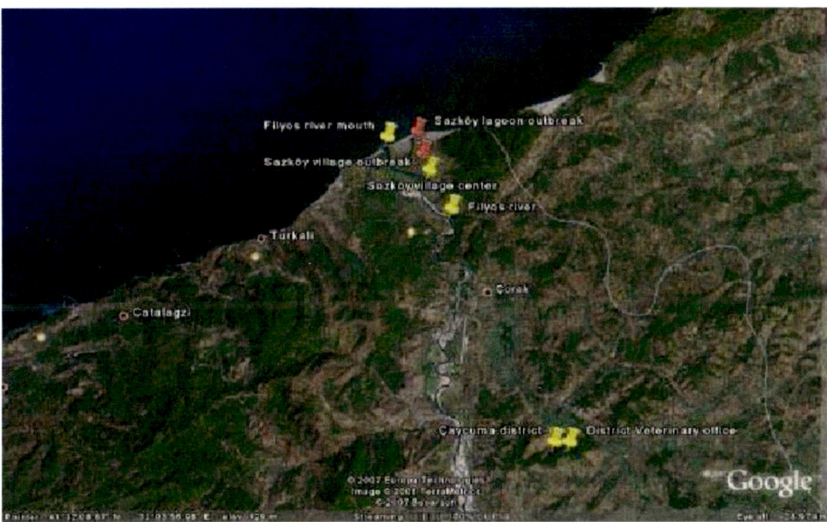


Google image-1: The location of Sazkoy village outbreak

*The map and image text used to illustrate the location of the Sazköy outbreak in the outbreak investigation report (Google Earth image by ©2007 Europa Technologies, ©2001 TerraMetrics and ©2007 Basarsoftin Van den Ende, Rinus and Ragip Bayraktar 2008 Sazkoy: 5.)*

Yellow pins with short texts compensate for the blurry picture by pointing out what is considered important: "Filyos river", "Filyos river mouth", "Sazköy village outbreak", "Sazköy lagoon outbreak", "Sazköy village center", "Çaycuma district" and "District veterinary office".[91] In other words, the map and the pins are emphasising the features textualized and included in the report; text and maps "realize capacities for the other"; they work together and strengthen each other.[92] This also involves keeping out what we saw was not included in the textualized versions of the outbreak places; the outbreak report does not tag the coop I saw at the entrance of the village or any other buildings related to poultry production.

---

[89] Asdal, Kristin 2012; Latour, Bruno and Steve Woolgar 1979

[90] Van den Ende, Rinus and Ragip Bayraktar 2008 Sazkoy: 5. Illustration text is also copied from the mentioned report.

[91] Van den Ende, Rinus and Ragip Bayraktar 2008 Sazkoy: 5

[92] Strathern, Marilyn 2003: 39

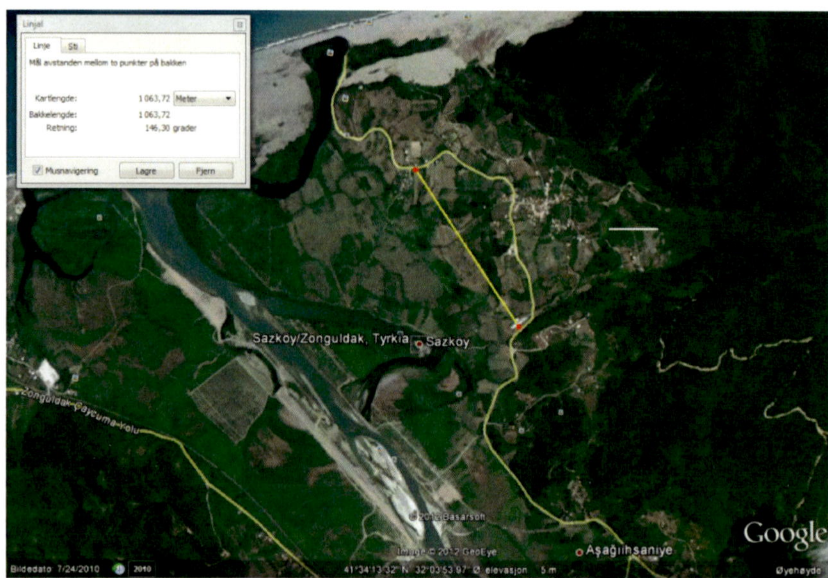


*Google Earth image selected and marked by me. The yellow line is added in order to highlight the spatial relation between the so-called infected house and garden (north) and the industrial poultry house (south). According to the textbox in the upper left corner, the direct distance between these two points is roughly 1064 meter. (Google Earth image by ©2012 Basarsoft)*

The picture at the top of the current page is a map I downloaded from Google Earth. When I made my own map of the outbreak place, I zoomed in on the 3-kilometre protection zone. At this scale, the narrow, long building housing the broilers fattened up by the village headman, *Muhtar*, and his family, is also visible. Because of my visit to Sazköy I know that this long building is a poultry house, and that it was operational during the outbreak. During my visit, I was also shown the outbreak house. Thus, I have added a line indicating the distance of 1063 meters between the outbreak house (north) and the coop (south). In this way, my map is including and making activities of this sector present at the outbreak place. While Filyos River, Sazköy lagoon and the Black Sea coast are also visible, they need to share the space with Muhtar's poultry house.

The AI project report also depicts Yörükler in Samsung Province, the second outbreak area, through a 'neutral' and 'natural' Google map (added below).[93] No pins point out important details on this map, except the outbreak

[93] Ivanov, Yanko and Ragip Bayraktat 2008 Yorukler: 7. Illustration text too is copied from the mentioned report.

place. According to my analysis of the textual enactment of this outbreak place in this report, the investigation team considered this area to be merely a wetland populated by wild birds and comprising a high population of backyard poultry. Accordingly, only wetlands and coastal lines appear on this map. From this distance, the map speaks for itself. Zooming brings in complexity though; for example, it is possible to see roads and buildings; hence, an area populated by humans, connected to rather than isolated from its surroundings, becomes visible.

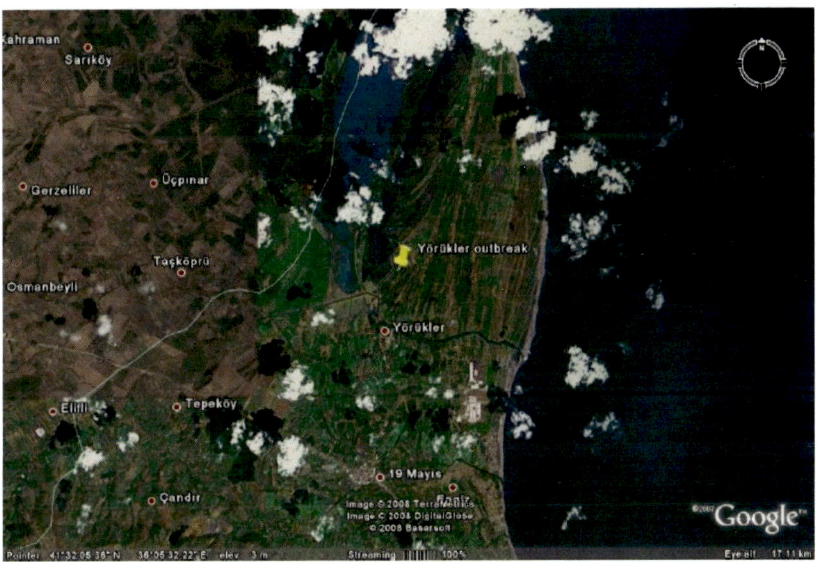


Google image-1: The location of Yorukler village where H5N1 outbreak was registered

*The map and image text used to illustrate the location of the Yörükler outbreak in the outbreak investigation report. Source: Google Earth image ©2008 TerraMetrics, © 2008 DigitalGlobe and ©2008 Basarsoft in Ivanov, Yanko and Ragip Bayraktat 2008 Yorukler: 7*

As depicted above, Samsun province (where the Yörükler and Aybeder outbreaks occurred) had the highest numbers of reported and confirmed cases during the large, countrywide wave of HPAI H5N1 in 2006. In the AI project report on the Yörükler outbreak, an additional Google Earth view of the province (added below), shows the number of "Confirmed Avian Influenza cases in Samsun province in 2006".[94] The text accompanying this map states that, "Samsun has clearly had the highest number of reported outbreaks of any province in both domestic and wild birds. Given the presence of important wetland sites, this may not seem surprising."[95]

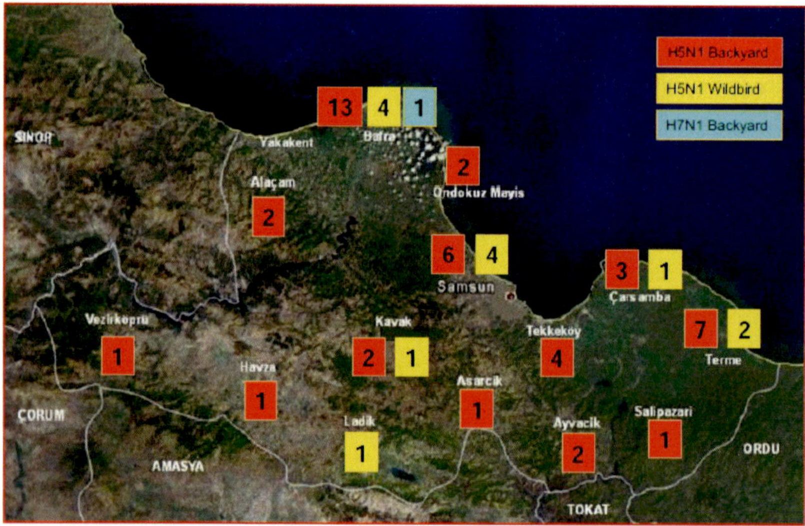


Fig 3: Confirmed Avian Influenza cases in Samsun province in 2006

*Ivanov, Yanko and Ragip Bayraktat 2008 Yorukler: 6.*

Neither the text nor the maps in this report give the poultry sector access to play a role, neither at the outbreak scene nor in the province more widely. I added one layer on the Google map of Samsun province in order to bring in this detail (my version of the Google map is added below). The red marks show the two confirmed outbreak areas in 2008; the yellow pins show the *districts* with commercial poultry production.[96] If each poultry house, feed mill, slaughterhouse and so on would have their own pin on this map, poultry related activities would of course be far more dominating.[97]

---

94 Ivanov, Yanko and Ragip Bayraktat 2008 Yorukler: 6. Illustration text too is copied from the mentioned report.

95 *Op. cit.*

96 Altındeğer, Mustafa and Burhan Hekimoğlu 201

97 The source from where I have found the poultry producing districts (*ibid.*) also provides numbers of various poultry produced in each district. This information is not included on my map.

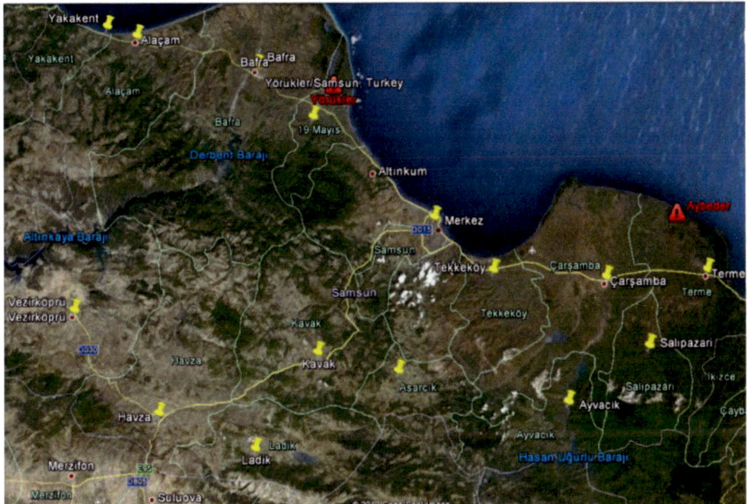


*Google earth map modified by me in order to include the two confirmed outbreak areas in 2008 (red signs) and districts with commercial poultry production (yellow pins). (Google Earth image © 2012 CNES Spot Image)*

## Looking further down at "wetlands" – a waterbody multiple

Wetlands, lakes and coastline are given a vital role in these outbreak investigation reports. This echoes my analysis in the previous chapter of how the avian influenza spread to Europe was inscribed in the Final version of the Global Strategy. Moreover, my analysis of the reports as well as of the strategy document showed how *waterbodies* come to equal *wild bird habitats.* Furthermore, wild, and possibly migratory, species are enacted as *threatening*, as they possess the ability of bringing avian influenza virus *into* the domestic sphere – the country or coop. Annemarie Mol's work on the multiple nature of *the* human body alerts us to the multiple nature of *the* waterbody, *the* wetland, or *the* delta.

For others situated in other scientific fields, wetlands may be something quite different. Within fields such as hydrology, fishery, environmental engineering or biology, several studies discuss the contamination of waterbodies as a result of insufficient or a total lack of treatment of wastewater *from* domestic sources, industry and agriculture included.[98] In this context, wild birds and other living organisms are enacted as *threatened*, rather than threatening. In a study of the water quality in Kızılırmak River for example, one of the large

98 On issues regarding industrial wastewater and domestic sewers see Okumus, Kerem 2002 I have previously addressed the issue of wastewater treatment related to the textile industry in Turkey (Madsen, Linda 2004)

rivers that contribute to enacting the Samsun province and the Yörükler outbreak place in the text studied above, the environmental engineers behind the study concluded the following:

Agricultural schemes within Kızılırmak River basin contributed to the deterioration of Kızılırmak River water quality. Major causes of concern are the fertilizers and chemicals. Run-off from agricultural schemes mostly contain chemical residues and fertilizers, which may pollute the water, and depending on loads may result in various hazards to the aquatic life and other lives depending on the river as a habitat and source of water supply.[99]

This particular study is enacting a connection between a Kızılırmak waterbody and domestic poultry where movement or contamination flow occurs in the opposite direction; from the domestic to the wild; contamination flow of the same waterbody is enacted as going *out to* the wild rather than *into* the domestic. This publication also draws attention to the "intensification of agriculture in the last decades [which] has been singled out as the most important non-point source of water pollution." In particular, this study is enacting, "runoff and erosion" from "fertilized agricultural lands" as a major concern for the quality of this specific waterbody. It is outside the scope of this project to investigate the relation between agricultural pollution and HPAI. To my current knowledge, no studies have investigated the possible virus contamination of waterbodies adjacent to H5N1 outbreak places in Turkey, despite the general agreement among experts that the virus could survive well in poultry manure and waterbodies.[100]

Poultry manure is addressed by the AI project, as the project was responsible for developing "Manual on Poultry Manure and Carcass Management."[101] I will suggest that the outbreak investigations formed part of the AI project's *emergency* management of the disease. Preparing the manure manual, on the other hand, formed part of the project's response to *emergent* matters, together with other matters such as improving the veterinary information system (Turkvet), exploring possibilities for compartmentalisation as a way to restructure poultry production, and implementing various training programs. Studying the outbreak investigation reports in this chapter shows that matters related

99 Gülfem Bakan, Hülya Böke Özkoç, Sevtap Tülek and Hüseyin Cüce 2010: 462. Regarding water quality in Lake Manyas, a waterbody that, in the outbreak report prepared by the Ministry of Agriculture and Rural Affairs (MARA/KKGM2005) was placed in relation to the initial outbreak in Turkey in 2005, please refer to Chapter 3 of this book and to my reference there to Karafistan, Aysel and Arik-Colakoglu, Fatma 2005.

100 See Fear, C. J. 2006

101 Aşkaroğlu, Haluk H., Yanko Ivanov and Ragip Bayraktar 2008

to poultry production have not been included in the inscription of the emergency situation of an outbreak; hence carcasses and manure both in the form of waste or fertilizer are absent from the waterbodies enacted in the outbreak investigation reports.

### Returning to mapping

If agricultural land fertilized with poultry manure, along with waterways that most likely contained untreated wastewater from units involved in poultry productions, such as factories, farms and households, had been be inscribed in the reports, this map, which re-contextualizes these outbreak places, would be far more complex. While these matters of concern are not included in the outbreak reports – they are neither inscribed by text nor by the maps – they are also absent when the topology of bio*in*security is being ordered and the context of outbreak places is enacted.

As demonstrated by studying the textual inscription of outbreak places, the fact that no outbreak was reported from commercial farms, together with a trust in the surveillance and reporting systems, works to justify that neither poultry houses or their produce ought to be included in the mapping of outbreak places. However, when materializing the context of outbreak place by maps, this outbreak investigation report reinforces both a trust in surveillance and reporting systems and a direction of virus flow – from the wild and *into the* domestic. This became apparent through my analysis of the strategy documents; in addition, Hinchliffe et al. have recently drawn attention to the implications of commonly perceived viral flows.[102]

The widespread outbreak in Samsun in 2006 was, as we saw on the map above, *naturalized*; The report stated that "[g]iven the presence of important wetland sites" it was not "surprising" that so many cases occurred in the province. As we saw when taking a close look at the tempo-spatial analysis above, a "propagating epidemic" was not identified in 2008, unlike in 2006. The *lack* of a propagating epidemic worked in 2008 as an argument against "poultry to poultry spread". When the 2006 outbreaks are made to contribute in the epidemiological discussion on the 2008 Yörükler outbreak, the former outbreaks display a propagating epidemic. This does not work in a way that suggests poultry to poultry spread, but on the contrary to make wild bird introduction a *natural* source of infection in 2006, in a double sense; the "*nature*" of this area is still the same – apparently it is an exclusively wild bird habitat – thus, it is natural that outbreaks would occur.

---

[102] Hinchliffe, Steve, John Allen, Stephanie Lavau, Nick Bingham and Simon Carter 2012

## Mapping avian influenza risk in Turkey

Natural features have also previously been mapped with the purpose to order avian influenza risk areas in Turkey. One country map that appears in several of the reports on outbreak investigations in Turkey – where otherwise no common standard apply to the maps used – is a country map displaying "Risk zone 1 to 3" (added below).[103] In the reports on the outbreaks in Sazköy, Yörükler and Esetçe, this map appears in the conclusion. The map serves to illustrate that "[avian influenza] H5N1 was introduced in backyard poultry" in villages that are "in [a] high risk zone identified by the [AI] project team".[104] No further information regarding what this risk evaluation is based on is provided in any of these reports. Nonetheless, the map works to support the conclusion that "[t]his outbreak might well serve to illustrate the fact that H5N1 can be introduced in Turkey by migratory birds."[105]

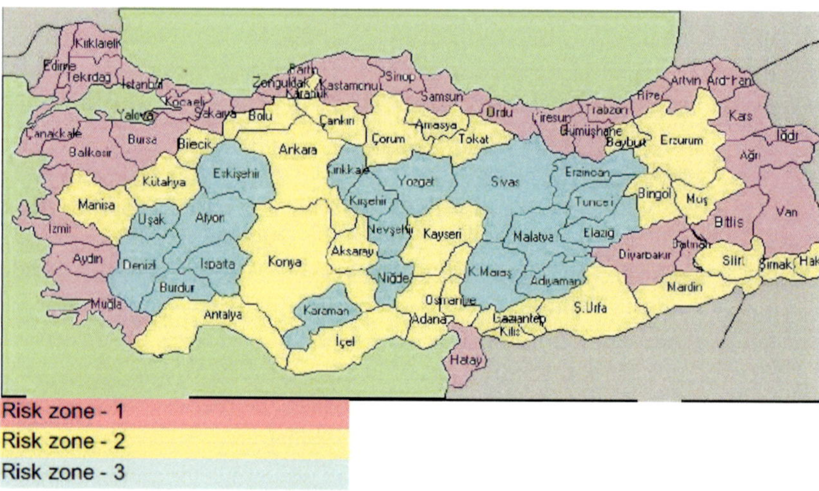


*Turkey avian influenza risk zone map. This is was found in Arik, Musa, Yanki Ivanov, Ragip Bayraktar and Marinus Van den Ende 2007: 51*

Searching for somewhere I could make some sense of what kind of sense this map is enacting, I ended up with the *Avian Influenza Surveillance Manual*

[103] Van den Ende, Rinus and Ragip Bayraktar 2008 Sazkoy: 11. Illustration text is also copied from the mentioned report.

[104] Van den Ende, Rinus and Ragip Bayraktar 2008 Sazkoy: 11; Ivanov, Yanko and Ragip Bayraktat 2008 Yorukler: 13; Van den Ende, Marinus and Ragip Bayraktar 2008 Esetce: 10

[105] *Op.cit.*

published by the AI project in 2007.[106] There I could see that the identification of risk zones in Turkey is based on a "tentative classification of 'eco-climatic zones'". It is the coastal and wetland habitats' proximity to migration routes that are transforming some provinces into red, high-risk zone-1 areas. "[B]ordering those in 'zone-1'" is a condition that gives an area the status of medium risk, while "[m]ountain areas without important lakes" and "central highlands" are relatively safe.[107]

In their study of wild bird surveillance in the UK, Steve Hinchliffe and Stephanie Lavau show how a report from a particular research project contribute to identifying "high-risk wild birds and at-risk places" by combining "information about the location and abundance of wild birds ( ... ) with data from the newly implemented national poultry register".[108] In this way, risk mapping in the UK and Turkey involves the inscription of different matters of concerns, as the UK risk map includes poultry. Furthermore, the mapping of avian influenza risk in Turkey is also quite different from other places, such as in Africa. A team working on the Early Detection Response and Surveillance of Avian Influenza in Africa project (EDRS-AIA), implemented by the International Livestock Research Institute (ILRI) in collaboration with African Union Interafrican Bureau for Animal Resources (AU/IBAR), published a document entitled *Risk Mapping for HPAI H5N1 in Africa – Improving surveillance for bird flu* (2010).This document brings several factors together that are weighted differently and are enacted by two different maps: one illustrates risk of *introduction to* Africa and the other illustrates risk of *spread in* Africa. Factors for introduction that are taken into account are "proximity to cross border roads", "proximity to water/wetlands", presence of three different migratory flyways, and proximity to ports. *Seven* factors for spread are taken into account: poultry density carries the most weight, followed by proximity to markets, primary roads, wetlands, secondary roads, irrigated areas and navigable rivers. In this way, the avian influenza risk maps for Africa inscribe a complex context for risk of introduction and spread of avian influenza. Viewed in relation to the Global Strategy, as analysed in Chapters 4 and 5, the risk maps for Africa inscribe some of the multiplicities of avian influenza; these maps are enacting avian influenza as possibly a poultry issue, an issue of economy and trade as well as a wildlife issue.

The Turkish avian influenza risk map only includes and inscribes factors related to wild birds, particularly migratory species and their habitats. Hence,

[106] Arik, Musa, Yanki Ivanov, Ragip Bayraktar and Marinus Van den Ende 2007: 51
[107] *Op.cit.*: 52
[108] Hinchliffe, Steve and Stephanie Lavau 2012: 263

this map is enacting a context for avian influenza risk in Turkey as being exclusively a matter of contact with wild birds. In this way, the entire Black Sea coastline is already ordered as a high risk zone, or Risk Zone 1 as the text on the map characterizes it, due to factors related to wild and possibly migratory birds. Thus, this map, or this version of avian influenza risk in Turkey, and the version of avian influenza introduction to these places enacted in the conclusion of the outbreak investigation reports, reinforce each other. Furthermore, the risk map and the joint mission's aggregated outbreak map displaying all the outbreaks (except the final outbreak which had yet to be reported) provide a context where it seems obvious to name this "wave of outbreaks" as "the Black Sea outbreak"; the maps work to convey the outbreaks on the Black Sea coastline, which had already been enacted as risky due to its association with wild birds, and in particular migratory birds entering these areas as they arrive, or come *into* Turkey.[109]

While cross-country borders and ports are matters of concern in the risk map on Africa, this is neither included on the risk map on Turkey nor in the mapping of particular outbreak places. For example, Samsung province, which had two outbreaks during this "wave", and which was hit hard the year before, has both an airport and a harbour with regular traffic between destinations in the Ukraine and Russia and other Black Sea harbours. Zonguldak, which is near to Sazköy, also has an international port, as does Bandırma, the city and commercial centre close to Manyas where the first outbreak in Turkey was reported in 2005. These three towns are also connected to the national railways. Furthermore, the proximity to the Greek border of the final outbreak in Esetçe was never included on this map and is not disturbing the conclusion that this was yet another outbreak with a wild bird source.

In a context where HPAI is commonly considered to evolve in situations of density, for example intensively raised poultry populations (as cited in the appendices to the Global Strategy in Chapter 4 of this book), it seems reasonable to include poultry density on a Turkish avian influenza risk map. This argument is further strengthened by the fact that both the UK risk map and the African avian influenza risk map include such data. On the African map, poultry density is considered the highest risk factor for spread within Africa. A map imaging "poultry unit density in Turkey" which can be found in an avian influenza market impact analysis and added below, may work to enact a different version of Turkey.[110] Here we see that the outbreaks in Sazköy, Yenicam

[109] On perceived direction of virus flow and implications thereof see Hinchliffe, Steve, John Allen, Stephanie Lavau, Nick Bingham and Simon Carter 2012

[110] Yalcin, Cengiz 2006 with reference to MARA 2006

and Konaçık (and also the above mentioned outbreak reported in Manyas in 2005) are well within the dark green areas with the highest numbers of poultry units. The Esetçe outbreak is positioned in a brighter green province indicating a lower number of units. Still, the outbreak location is close to the border of the neighbouring province, which is coloured dark green and thus enacted as having a high poultry density on this map. According to this map, the outbreaks in Samsung province and Sinop province do not fall into risk areas when they are enacted in accordance to poultry unit density.[111]

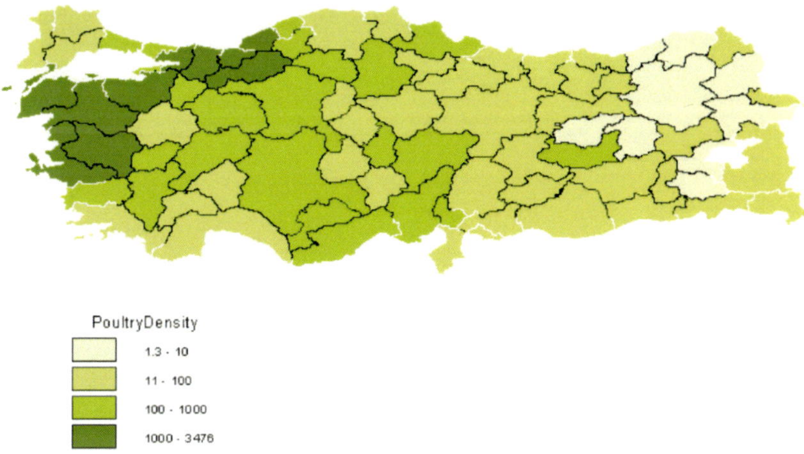


*"Map of poultryunit density in Turkey Source: MARA 2006" in Yalcin, Cengiz 2006*

Returning to the avian influenza risk map for Turkey, and the map providing an overview of the so-called 2006 Black Sea outbreaks, the only features that are inscribed are coast or waterbody outbreak places. Thus, the only spatial relations these maps enact are the connection between outbreaks and the coast or a waterbody, and the spatial relations between the outbreaks. Other information related to what is in-between, matters of human geography, such as roads and other infrastructure or industry/production, are not included on the risk map or the country maps studied in the section above. These factors are not inscribed when the avian influenza risk in Turkey are mapped nor in the reports on particular outbreak situations.

In order to contextualize these outbreaks and relevant aspects of my fieldwork (at the beginning of this chapter), I could have selected a map from the

111 Among the obvious problems with this map, it should be noted that it portrays provinces and actual numbers of poultry units; thus, it does not mention poultry density within a unit

joint mission report that "show location of the outbreaks".[112] All I needed to do was add a mark to indicate the Esetçe outbreak. Using a different map to present my fieldwork is a way to connect this chapter with Chapter 2, given that the same map is used to offer a more general methodological presentation of this book. Furthermore, I found it necessary to display these places in the introduction of this chapter; however, analytically, the joint mission outbreak map fits in here. Therefore, I decided to use these two different maps, which are imaging the same place.

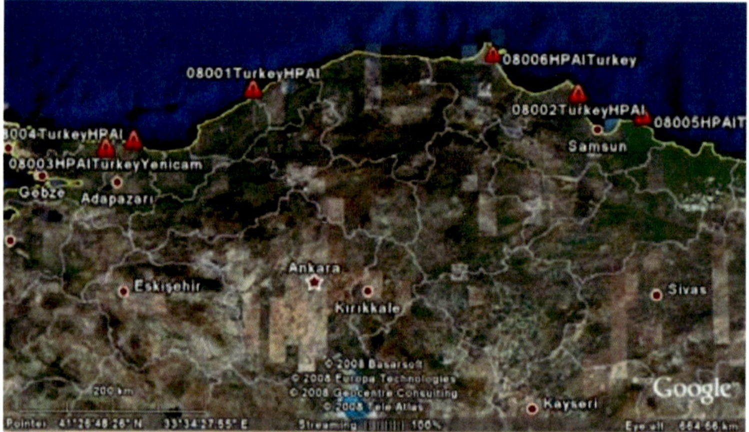


*The 2008 outbreaks mapped by the AI project. (Google Earth image by ©2008 Basarsoft, ©2008 Europa Technologies, ©2008 Geocentre consulting and 2005 Tele Atlas in Newman, Scott H., Nick Honhold, Javier Sanz-Alvarez and Kiraz Erciyas 2008: 12)*

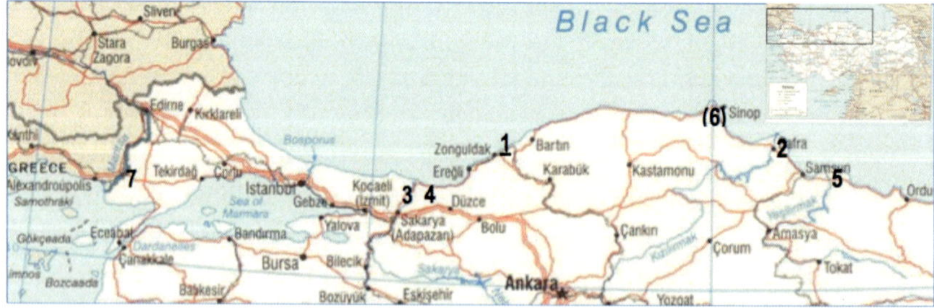


*My alternative mapping of the 2008 outbreaks. The source of original map it the U.S. Central Intelligence Agency (2006) but the map has been edited by here for the purpose of this project.*

---

[112] Newman, Scott H., Nick Honhold, Javier Sanz-Alvarez and Kiraz Erciyas 2008: 12

By oscillating between these two maps, or these two different versions of the same outbreak places, we can se that they do however, realize capacities of each other:[113] The map I chose for inscribing places for fieldwork makes me realize another spatial relation; it makes me realize how the joint mission map contributes to disarticulating alternatives.[114] The relation between outbreaks and the Black Sea coastline is still present on my fieldwork map. However, on this map another line also connects these outbreak places: the thin, red line indicating the Black Sea *road*. The road follows the coastline but turns inland just by the two outbreaks in Sakarya (marked as 3 and 4), which also happened further inland.

Studying how maps contribute to ordering and enacting these particular outbreak places, and the relation between them and to other matters of concern enables us to see how this involves inclusion and exclusion. Moreover, maps enact particular presences and disarticulate alternatives in ways that both reduce complexities and enable conclusions, but which also contribute to enacting avian influenza as*a* particular issue: a wild bird issue.[115] However, how is this conclusion being stabilized and secured? The tool for doing so will be analysed in the following section.

## Tools for ordering III: Copy/Paste- tool

The most obvious effect of copy/paste-technology is efficiency. Needless to say – although still important for academics to keep in mind – the management of on-going outbreak events demands action, and not least the reporting and publication of results, at a different speed than for example a long term research project. As we saw in the previous chapter, the first outbreak of HPAI H5N1 detected in Turkey in October 2005 was subject to rapid epidemiological inquiries. The source of infection was determined fast enough for the conclusions to contribute to moving avian influenza towards being a wild bird issue at the time of publication of the Final version of the Global Strategy one month later, in November 2005.[116] Copying/pasting text from one document or report to another is first of all time saving, labour efficient and a very useful aid when working under time pressure. However, does it also have other implications or effects? In the previous chapters, which focussed on avian influenza strategies,

[113] Strathern, Marilyn 1991, with reference to Haraway, Donna 1985

[114] Strathern, Marilyn 1991 and Moser, Ingunn 2008

[115] The implications of the use of numbers and maps in relation to avian influenza is discussed by Scoones, Ian and Paul Forster 2008

[116] FAO, OIE and WHO 2005 Nov.

I found that text which moves and keeps its shape can both influence and become influenced by its context.[117] Following one particular sentence, I now aim to see how this text contributes to ordering the avian influenza reality, and how it contributes to enacting context and how context may influence the content of this text.

## Inscribing exclusions, enacting absence and removing complexities

> By extensive inquiry, no evidence could be found for introduction of the virus by movements of animals or people or trade in live poultry or poultry products, or by gifts of the same.[118]

I encountered this sentence in the Sazköy outbreak investigation report and wondered: This seems familiar. Have I not read this before? Yes, I had indeed read it before. A very similar sentence appears in the common investigation report on the Batman[119] and Diyarbakır outbreaks report that I had read the year before:

> By extensive inquiry no evidence could be found for introduction of the virus by purchase of live poultry or poultry products, or by gifts of the same.[120]

This clear, precise and conclusive sentence stands out among the rest for its strictly formulated language; it is specific at the same time as it excludes a wide range of possible sources of introduction in a way that limit complexities and removes uncertainty. The Batman and Diyarbakır were the first reported cases of HPAI H5N1 investigated by the AI project. These outbreaks were reported shortly after the AI project began and one year before the Black Sea outbreaks. The sentence appears early on in the report on the Sazköy outbreak. There it contributes to enacting the context for the outbreak in a way that enables the result of the investigation; the report excludes domestic poultry as a possible source of introduction, thus it establishes certain conditions that set the grounds for the events that could possibly have taken place.[121] The sentence efficiently clears the path for the theories that follow; the rest of the section is dedicated to wild birds, and several possibilities for how wild birds may have introduced the

---

[117] Law, John and Annemarie Mol 2001

[118] Van den Ende, Rinus and Ragip Bayraktar 2008 Sazkoy: 8

[119] In response to my caring proof reader and in order to avoid potential confusion among other readers unfamiliar with the southeastern parts to Turkey: Batman is the true name of a town close to the border to Iran –not a result of unwanted auto-correction.

[120] Honhold, Nick and Ragip Bayraktar 2007 Diyarbakir and Batman

[121] Asdal Kristin 2012

virus to the village are presented. The report does not conclude on the source of introduction, but it carefully formulates that there is "overall evidence on wild bird *involvement* in this outbreak".[122] In extension to this, the report calls for follow-up studies on the role of wild birds, in particular migratory ones. In this way, the wild bird focus is also immediately followed up by the AI project; the project continues on the same path as the Ministry of Agriculture, which pointed out that wild birds were the source of introduction for the infected turkeys in Manyas during the initial 2005 outbreak in Turkey.[123]

During the weeks following the first reported case in Batman, 17 more cases were detected.[124] The investigations that followed concluded that wild birds were the probable *source*, but that "*spread* ha[d] been through fomites".[125] In this latter report, which included all 18 cases, the problem of identifying where the virus actually hit first, the so-called *primary case*, was recognized. It remained uncertain if the virus had already circulated to other places at the time of the so so-called *index case*, the first case detected.[126] The remote position of the first reported case, together with presence of wild birds, on-going hunting activity, and, last but not least, the "'*absence of [... ]domestic poultry source",* contributed to allowing the first detected case to retain its status as the primary case.[127] Thus, wild birds kept their role as the possible *source* of infection even when more outbreaks were detected and reported. Crucially, as the virus was identified at several places in this area, these incidents were ordered in a way that made *these 18 cases together enact one outbreak*. Thus, in the Batman and Diyarbakır outbreak, *spread* and the epidemic threat became a major concern that partly overshadowed the importance of *source* of introduction, which was recognized as being surrounded by uncertainties. The common report on this one outbreak, involving 18 cases, states that "[t]o an extent [the source] is not important in that it is spread that makes epidemics."[128]

---

[122] Honhold, Nick and Ragip Bayraktar 2007 Diyarbakir and Batman: p. E2, *emphasis added*. In an e-mail attached to this outbreak report the epidemiologist shares his updates on the situation in Turkey with an unnamed receiver, apparently his FAO colleagues. Here he states more directly that "the source is likely to be wildbirds" (p. E4).

[123] MARA/KKGM 2005. This has also been discussed, especially in Chapter 3 of this volume.

[124] Bayraktar, Ragıp 2007. In addition, one case was detected in wild birds (*ibid.*).

[125] Bayraktar Ragip 2007: 6 *emphasis added*

[126] Bayraktar Ragip 2007: 7 *emphasis added*

[127] Bayraktar Ragip 2007: 7 *emphasis added* See also abovementioned e-mail where the epidemiologist, Nick Honhold shares his updates on the situation in Turkey with an unnamed receiver (apparently his FAO colleagues) (Honhold, Nick and Ragip Bayraktar 2007: p E4)

[128] Bayraktar Ragip 2007: 8: *emphasis added*

Returning to the 2008 Black Sea outbreaks, the so-called temporal analytical epidemiology at work in the investigations of these outbreaks contributes to ordering them in a way that makes them vitally different from the Batman and Diyarbakir outbreak, in that they were defined as "a series of separate introductions". Thus, here we had *seven outbreaks,* and not a propagating epidemic like in Batman and Diyarbakır the year before.[129] In this way, *introduction* becomes the major concern rather than spread, as was the case in the Batman and Diyarbakır outbreak. This again, cleared the way for that particular sentence to appear in several outbreak reports. This sentence is only about a possible *source of introduction.*

The sentence was slightly adjusted as it reoccurred in the report on the outbreak in Sazköy. From excluding "purchase of live poultry or poultry products" in the initial Batman case, the sentence was extended to *articulate alternatives* for spread and introduction generally assumed to be the most important – that is the "movements of animals or people" – in a way that also *excludes* these alternatives.[130] By excluding any possible alternatives, the sentence contributes to enacting a context for virus introduction where only wild birds remain present.

The sentence also appears in the AI project's report on the investigation of the Yörükler outbreak, which was the second reported incidence in the 2008 Black Sea outbreak. Directly copied from the Sazköy report, the text assures the reader that,

> By extensive inquiry, no evidence could be found for introduction of the virus by movements of animals or people or trade in live poultry or poultry products, or by gifts of the same.[131]

And finally, in the report on the last confirmed outbreak in Esetçe, situated close to the Greek border, the sentence does what it can to stabilize the fact, that:

> By extensive inquiry, no evidence could be found for introduction of the virus by movements of animals or people or trade in live poultry or poultry products, or by gifts of the same.[132]

---

[129] Newman, Scott H., Nick Honhold, Javier Sanz-Alvarez and Kiraz Erciyas 2008: 12

[130] See FAO, OIE and WHO 2005 May; 2005 Nov; FAO 2008 and Chapter 4 and 5 of this book. The way the alternatives are articulated and included but still excluded with reference to "extensive inquiry", alerts us to the nuances between *exclusion* on the one hand, and *lack of inclusion* or *disarticulation* These rhetorical means deserves further attention; unfortunately it is not possible for me to develop this further within the frame of this project.

[131] Ivanov, Yanko and Ragip Bayraktar 2008 Yorukler: 11

[132] Van den Ende, Marinus and Ragip Bayraktar 2008 Esetce: 9

All the way, or every time it shows up, the sentence works as a tool to exclude elements that may disturb the conclusion, which in all cases point to a wild bird *source* of infection.[133]

So, when turning around and reflect on the current section of this book chapter and the *extensive inquiry* conducted here it is timely to ask: in what way has the context changed since the sentence contributed in the Batman report, and in what way does the changing context influence the sentence itself and the realities it is textualizing? In Batman and Diyarbakır, *spread* was of major concern. On the other hand, the investigation reports on the Black Sea outbreaks ordered the outbreaks in a way that made them all *primary cases*, thus they were all in need of a *source of introduction*, and together they acted as "a series of introductions". The reports on the 2008 Black Sea outbreaks thus provide a strategic place for theories of introduction to evolve and re-evolve. When this sentence is at work in the reports on the Black Sea outbreaks, the sentence not only works as a tool for wild birds to be *involved*, such as in Batman; rather, here it contributes to paving the way for what would be characterized as "one of the *clearest and most direct examples to date, of introduction of infection* to domestic poultry from wild birds."[134]

In addition, since the *source of introduction* is now over and over again the issue in this "series of introductions", there is also room for the sentence to reappear over and over again. The way these cases of infection are enacted as being of a repetitive nature is important in the stabilization of facts. In one of the last documents published by the AI project team shortly before the project was completed, they summarize the following:

> Although circumstantial evidence for the wild bird role in HP H5N1 transmission abounds, clear proof is still lacking. The fact that since its appearance, no HP H5N1 virus has been detected in swab samples collected from over 500,000 waterfowl [worldwide I assume] has raised controversy about the role of birds in cross-border transmission of the virus and is used as an argument against it. However, analysis of past HP H5N1 outbreaks in Turkey has *time and again* pointed at the role of wild birds in their origin.[135]

Despite uncertainty, lack of evidence, controversy, and not least complexity, outbreak investigations have "time and again pointed at the role of wild

[133] For a similar point see Steve Hincliffe and Stephanie Lavau (2013) who state "[t]ruth is not conveyed by reference but by continual renewal on a message".

[134] Newman, Scott H., Nick Honhold, Javier Sanz-Alvarez and Kiraz Erciyas 2008:13, *emphasis added*

[135] AI project 2008: 6, *emphasis added*.

birds".[136] I will argue that the context in which the sentence is used, namely where introduction has become the major concern, together with the repetitive use of the sentence, makes the sentence more powerful. As my analysis has shown earlier in this chapter, the repetitive reference to wild birds has also been accompanied by the repetitive exclusion of other factors relevant for the prevention and control of avian influenza; this is precisely what this sentence contributes to.

## Trapped in the "missing middle"

Initially, this chapter suggested that outbreak investigations in Turkey might be seen as an attempt to fill the "missing middle" like Scoones called for; ideally, outbreak investigations should provide epidemiological knowledge and take into account local variations related to infectious diseases and epidemics, and thereby correct inadequate demands from above.[137] Scoones points out that what he sees as a vital problem and obstacle for disease response is that authoritative knowledge "is created at the top through particular types of expertise".[138] Furthermore, according to Scoones, this knowledge is often "codified in simple models and plans which do not accept uncertainty, ignorance or complexity".[139] A crucial question is then, to what extent are these problems overcome by filling the "missing middle" with sense makers on the ground, or, in this case, with experts carrying out outbreak investigations?

### Ordering and separation: Enacting mobile and immobile versions of outbreak places

Through detailed analysis, this chapter has shown how, despite the complex nature of transboundary infectious diseases, the outbreak investigation reports have contributed to ordering these places in a way that provides "strong evidence that the 2008 outbreak has a wild bird source," and that introduction happened "most likely via hunting practises". Furthermore, by studying the 2008 Black Sea outbreaks, I have seen how these have become "the clearest examples of a wild bird source of H5N1 HPAI in domestic poultry to date."[140]

---

136 *Op. cit.*

137 See FAO, OIE and WHO 2005 May; 2005 Nov; Scoones, Ian 2010

138 Scoones, Ian 2010: 215

139 *Op.cit.*

140 Newman, Scott H., Nick Honhold, Javier Sanz-Alvarez and Kiraz Erciyas 2008. There are no page numbers but the text is taken from the "Overall conclusion".

Moreover, my analysis shows that the "strong evidence" and the "clearest examples" depend on separation and of keeping matters apart.

Throughout this chapter, we have seen how investigation reports on specific outbreaks among backyard poultry in Turkey in 2008 contribute to *separating* wild birds from other possible sources of virus introduction through processes of lack of inclusion and exclusion. The tools for outbreak investigation reporting are working to order complexities; they work as means for inclusion, exclusion and separation. Through processes of ordering, outbreak places are made governable. In response to Scoones' call for room for complexity, my analysis has demonstrated that complexities are not allowed to remain complex here "on the ground" at the Turkish outbreak places either. Law advocates the co-existence of several order*s*, and writes that the nightmare of modernity is "the idea that there is a *single* order".[141] My analysis has shown how, in order to appear clear, the conclusions of the outbreak investigations are dependent on just *one single mode of ordering*. It can be argued that producing conclusions is necessary to justify interventions for disease control and to meet the demands of what Forester and Scoones refer to as "the contemporary mantra" of "evidence-based policy" of international governance of infectious diseases.[142]

As my analysis has shown, when various matters were excluded from being inscribed in a report, this does not necessarily imply that these matters were not being addressed. According to my informants, at the very least the coop involved in commercial production that I asked specific about, that is, the coop in Sazköy, was checked for H5N1. No infection had been detected among these birds. Hence, instead of being made part of the outbreak in a way that would turn the chickens into carcasses, or poultry culled as part of disease control, and thus included in the report, these chickens were excluded. Consequently, they were allowed to continue living; the only difference was the poultry were subjected to stricter surveillance and they were slaughtered at the age of 37 days rather than 45 days.[143] Moreover, manure and carcasses in general were a matter of concern in a manual created as part of the AI project's work on disease *prevention* and distributed among the commercial poultry sector. In

---

[141] Law, John 1994: 2. Also see Chapter 1 of this volume

[142] Scoones, Ian and Paul Forster 2008; Stirling, Andy C. and Ian Scoones 2009

[143] This one coop mentioned here by me, but absent from the report, on Sazköy, Zonguldak Province (Van den Ende, Rinus and Ragip Bayraktar 2008 Sazkoy). In Yenicam, Sakarya province one farm is, as mentioned, included in the report, which then ensures that no infection was detected there (Newman, Scott H., Nick Honhold, Javier Sanz-Alvarez and Kiraz Erciyas 2008).

relation to disease *response* – when the disease had occurred and outbreak places were inscribed in the reports – such matters were either simply not included, or they were excluded, for example by the specific sentence I follow when analysing the effect of what I call the copy/paste tool. The matter was handled separately.

How this separation was made possible became visible when I oscillated between the two versions of introduction and spread; one enacted by wild birds and another by commercial poultry. This made me realise how the criteria for access to the outbreak investigation reports differ for domestic and wild birds. Moreover, the analysis also shows how a presumption of well-working reporting together with an idea of controllability of the sector enabled topographic models that contributed to exclude commercial poultry as well as other humanly induced mechanisms for introduction and spread. Interestingly, my analysis has shown how simple topographic models as an epidemiologic tool for tracing introduction and spread enact an image of outbreak places and the space in between them as a transparent and complete whole. This version differs from what we saw when studying the specificities of individual cases or outbreaks; then, reporting of clinical signs of disease by poultry owners appeared to be accidental rather than common routine in line with a well working notification system. The AI project's work addressed the shortcomings of and the urgent need to improve both surveillance and reporting of suspected cases of avian influenza. They were carrying out training programs for the purpose of improving disease surveillance in poultry, and they produced publications that stressed the importance of prompt and sufficient compensation for reporting of suspected cases of avian influenza.[144] Significantly, these matters are handled separately; they are not included in the outbreak investigation reports.

### Emergency and the emergent: Reducing or embracing complexity

All these various measures which I have only briefly touched upon in this chapter – ones related for example to manure and carcass handling, surveillance, systems for compensation, and also the development of an veterinary information system (TURKVET) – show how the AI project – the *Technical Assistance to Avian Influenza Preparedness and Response Project in Turkey* – has addressed complexities in order to strengthen the preconditions of the Turkish Government for handling the *emergent* problems associated with emerging disease. In the context of dealing with an emergency, as when an outbreak or a

[144] An overview of the AI project, activities *Workpackages* is still (04.08.2014) available on http://www.prwatson.co.uk/TR_06_AI_SV/English/start.htm

wave of outbreaks has to be handled, reducing complexity makes the *emergency* governable. This is achieved by ordering work through a process of inclusion and exclusion; it involves making some matters absent and others present in the reports – but as was clear in this case, it also involved taking care of matters that remain absent from the report.

Hence, at the very same time – in the time of emergency – an outbreak is ordered, inscribed, materialized and made mobile in the form of reports. These reports contribute to filling the missing middle; ongoing situations of *emergency* are textualized and answer to the *emergent* need for knowledge to improve preparedness for future events. This is a vital moment of friction as times, matters and spaces interfere and lead to something new; in the form of a report, outbreak places are being de-contextualized but also re-contextualized. While matters inscribed in the outbreak investigation reports are departing from the outbreak place, and move on to contributing to policy making and the global governance of infectious disease, other matters of concern remain at the outbreak site; these latter may involve flexible solutions and improvisation, just as well as specific procedures – but they do not make it across the "missing middle"; they do not reach "the top" in a way that enable them to contribute, with their presence, to policy development. Nevertheless, the absence of Muhtar's poultry house, of the Turkish "lifestock revolution", of highways, airports and harbours and of other complex matters have effect: Their absence is making the wild bird theories strong, hence justifies particular biopolitical interventions.

## Re-thinking relations between exclusion and marginalization

Studying outbreak investigation reports has made it apparent that here, it is not those commonly assumed to be marginalized, namely the wild birds, backyard poultry and their owners, that are excluded.[145] Rather, it is the commercial poultry sector, commonly assumed to represent strong and well-organized actors and a locomotive for agricultural development, which is being excluded. Moreover, while feminist scholars of technoscience tend to see a mutual relationship between the marginalized and the excluded, the analysis of this chap-

[145] Backyard poultry owners are also referred to as "the rural poor" in a wide range of FAO publications. Even though this is outside the scope of this project, it is timely to emphasize that the category of "backyard poultry owners" is as heterogeneous as any other. While few if any are becoming economic wealthy from being a backyard poultry owner in Turkey, backyard poultry hold is practiced by rich as well as poor families due to the birds' value as pets and because meat from "self grown" chickens is regarded as tastier.

ter suggests the opposite; that in relation to disease outbreaks, inclusion implies marginalization. The way wild birds have been included makes them *the* (only!) possible source of infection – they have become agents of bio*in*security. Moreover, "the free ranging nature" of backyard poultry has been enacted as a bio*in*secure practice due to their possible contact with wildlife and their scavenging habits. By being excluded, matters remain absent when the topology of bio*in*security is enacted – they are secured and remain biosecure.

The different standards applied to wild birds compared to other possible sources of infection, in terms of identifying them as the source, further illustrates how the relation between inclusion and empowerment cannot be taken for granted. Furthermore, by being included in the report and hence becoming part of the official eradication program, backyard poultry were subjected to culling. Exclusion, on the other hand, protected commercial poultry from this fate. Moreover, a market analysis demonstrates that avian influenza outbreaks have a negative impact on the poultry market.[146] Market concerns emphasise the importance of keeping the commercial poultry sector separated from the avian influenza issue in order to avoid "market shock".[147]

By the commercial poultry sector being left absent from the inscribed, mobile versions of outbreak places, *and* by these events being enacted as a wild birds- and backyard poultry issue, the commercial sector remains secure; the way outbreak places are enacted in the investigation reports prevent this sector from being associated with the matters of bio*in*security. Moreover, the improvisations, ad-hoc solutions, adaptation and fluidities that make eradication work, do not make it through the missing middle – it is not mentioned in the outbreak investigation reports and does not travel to the international community. And just this might make us scrutinize the role of outbreaks investigation reports in filling the missing middle: directly translating an emergency, in the form of outbreak investigation reports, into emergent plans for disease control may well contribute to what Hinchliffe refers to as the insecurities of biosecurity.[148]

---

[146] Yalcin, Cengiz 2006

[147] *Ibid*; See also Ivanov, Yanko 2007

[148] Hinchliffe, Steve 2013 in Dobson, Andrew, Kezia Barker and Sarah L. Taylor (Eds.)

# 7. Arriving

"[N]ear the Yörükler [outbreak] site", "a common buzzard, *buteo buteo*", was reportedly "found moribund and euthanized" by a team of wild life experts and ornithologist conducting the *Joint EU-FAO Avian Influenza Outbreak Investigation Mission,* a mission I referred to in the previous chapter as the FAO-EU joint mission.[1] Arriving at the end of this book, this dead – though arguably still highly vital – buzzard will assist me in drawing together the major findings presented throughout this work. I do not intend to position myself on the back of this buzzard so that it can take me high up in the sky and bring me to the point where I would have the birds-eye view of this project or of the avian influenza issue, neither literally nor metaphorically. Rather than creating an overview and rather than aiming for generalizations, in this final chapter I will draw on the buzzard's keen sight. Hawk-eyed, or with a buzzard's vision, I set out to clarify the main findings of this study of avian influenza in Turkey and beyond. This dead but mobile buzzard will contribute to highlighting the outcomes of distinct ethnographic moments, illuminating some whole images (which are not to be confused with an image of a whole), pointing out some ponds within ponds, and emphasising crucial results of attending to specificities, as I have done throughout this book. In this way, we remain close to the analytical insights that have guided this work.[2]

In order to study the specificities of avian influenza, three interrelated approaches have been central throughout in this study; through a processual, performative and relational approach I have examined the *becoming* of avian influenza; I have studied how avian influenza is being enacted and performed through processes and relations. In this way, I have challenged the traditional biomedical and technical approaches to disease control, which are commonly operating from a normative stance where the problem or issue is taken for granted or is defined based on pre-conceived norms in ways that request particular interventions to regain "normality".[3] By studying various processes and relations through which avian influenza is enacted, I have traced how avian in-

1 Newman, Scott, Nick Honhold, Javier Sanz-Alvarez and Kiraz Erciyas 2008: 4

2 Law, John 2002a 2004a; Strathern, Marilyn 2004; See also Asdal, Kristin 2014; Mol, Annemarie 2002 Moser, Ingunn 2005. As discussed in Chapter 2, the concept of 'ethnographic moments' are used in this volume in accordance with Anna Tsing's (2005) definition.

3 Please refer to Chapter 1 for a further discussion.

fluenza is multiple[4] and heterogeneous[5]. Moreover, my analysis has also shown how one version – a particular version of avian influenza as a wild bird issue where wild birds introduce the virus *to* domestic birds, and where backyard poultry are considered an insecure form of life due to their "free ranging nature" and contact with the wild – has gained strength, at the cost of other versions. A more detailed *re-view* of how this has occurred and its implications for governance will be presented in this concluding chapter.

A final matter of concern that has guided this work, and which should be highlighted before discussing the major results of the analysis, is*mobility*:[6] for example, mobility within the composition of the H5N1 virus genome as it changes from low to high pathogenic;[7] the mobility of the virus between species and space making it a zoonotic and transboundary matter of concern and a "global threat" to animals, humans, and the economy;[8] the mobility of concepts and strategies for disease governance; the mobility and mobilization of analytical notions; and mobility within and beyond the empirical field.[9] As will soon be apparent, despite – or rather because of – the buzzard's miserable condition, it works well to seize some key points regarding mobility.

In terms of mobility, how may this research project, which engages with past disease outbreaks as well as recent and less recent theoretical contributions, influence the direction of future research within and beyond the academic field of STS? Moreover, how might it intervene in disease governance for the future? Finally, how does my particular, but not exclusive, focus on Turkey contribute to realizing "global" matters of concern, such as avian influenza, in a new way?

Four major outcomes of this project should be emphasised. Firstly, this study has shown *how* avian influenza is multiple and heterogeneous, and how the mode in which it is enacted (or not) has biopolitical implications. Secondly, it addresses the importance of insecurity for security and argues that

---

4 Mol, Annemarie 2002

5 Law, John 1986

6 Among the central resources this work is drawing on are: Law, John 1986; Law John and Annemarie Mol 2001; Latour, Bruno 1999; Asdal, Kristin 2007.

7 Please refer to the discussion on emergence in Chapter 4. See also Chapter 5 on the role of wild birds in the spread, and how both virus and wild bird theories "spread". Bio(in)security, as discussed in Chapter 3, also deals with mobility at several levels.

8 Please refer to the discussions on poultry, human health and the economy in Chapter 4, where I also discuss how concepts travel (see especially the section on poultry issues and the discussion on "backyard poultry").

9 Chapters 1 and 2 provide the most thorough theoretical and methodological discussions related to mobility; an overall goal has been to *add* analytical approaches throughout the book, including new but related resources in each chapter.

bio*in*security deserves direct attention in a symmetrical way to biosecurity. Thirdly, my analysis contributes to rethinking how to understand global-local relations. Thinking in terms of *connecting locals* has proven useful for overcoming hierarchical top-down approaches and it invites processual and relational approaches through which one can trace the becoming of avian influenza – as well as any issues that takes the form of something "global". As a fourth and final major point, by drawing attention to how ordering complexity involves inclusion and exclusion as well as the making of absence and presence, the analyses has shown how the relation between exclusion and marginalization on the one hand, and inclusion and empowerment on the other hand, should not be taken for granted.

In order to capture these major interrelated empirical and analytical points, I will utilize the raptor's ability to seize and take hold; *with* this particular buzzard, found at the location and in the context where this book ends, I aim to re-view my major findings. This dead buzzard is *energizing*. Thus it reminds us not to take capacities for granted. I will argue that this deceased bird has the power to engage, arouse and excite. Furthermore, despite its condition, or perhaps because of it, this buzzard is mobile and able to move far beyond the Turkish wetlands. I aim to empower the main arguments of this book as I let these arguments follow and interact with this energetic, dead buzzard on its journey from the Turkish wetlands into the "global" biopolitical agenda.

## Wetlands are turning into real-world laboratories and a moribund buzzard is turning into a "significant finding"

Because this bird received the status as "a significant finding" by the FAO-EU joint mission, it is reasonable to assume that this "moribund buzzard" aroused the interest of the team who found it. In order to recapitulate how this dying bird turned into "a significant finding" in the first place, I will re-draw the context within which it was found. The report on the FAO-EU joint mission characterises the mission as a global, historical event:

> This *was the first time globally*, that a mission attempted to conduct concurrent poultry outbreak investigations coupled with wild bird census activities, monitoring for dead wild birds, and wild bird capture and sampling.[10]

How did this happen? How did, as this text says, outbreak investigations in Turkey come to be "coupled with" various "wild bird census activities"? As

[10] Newman, Scott and Nick Honhold, Javier Sanz-Alvarez, Kiraz Erciyas 2008: 3, *italics added*

my study of the Global Strategy has shown, the role of wild birds in relation to avian influenza was a major matter of concern for the international community. This was already apparent in the draft version of the Global Strategy, which was published before the virus spread beyond Asia. As my analysis of the official investigations of particular outbreaks in Turkey in Chapter 3 shows, this initial outbreak, reported in backyard poultry, were placed in relation to wild birds rather than commercial poultry production or any other possible source of infection. The outbreak report, published by the Turkish Ministry of Agriculture and Rural Affairs (MARA), concluded that wild birds were *a likely source of infection*. Just as importantly, wild birds were *the only likely* source mentioned.

However, it was more to this than introduction to Turkey. The way virus introduction was enacted, as a wild bird issue, also came to imply that long distance spread from Asia to Turkey, *through wild bird migration*, was possible. This triggered the already latent international interest in the issue. As my analysis in Chapter 5 details, the ordering of the initial outbreaks in Turkey and a few other European countries, and the way these were inscribed in the updated, Final, version of the Global Strategy, contributed to moving avian influenza towards becoming a wild bird issue. Moreover, this was happening in a way that also expanded the role of wild birds, from being local reservoirs to being long distance transporters of the HPAI virus.

When epidemiological investigations of two outbreaks, reported close to the Black Sea coast in the north-western part of Turkey during the early months of 2008, concluded that "[t]his outbreak might well serve to illustrate the fact that H5N1 can be introduced in Turkey by migratory birds", villages were not only transformed into outbreak places. These villages and certain surrounding areas were enacted as particular versions of wetlands and as potential real-world laboratories.[11] The reports from the initial two outbreaks recommended that "[f]ollow up studies should be conducted ( … ), to produce convincing scientific evidence for the role of wild birds in virus spreading".[12] In an email, sent from the FAO to Turkish authorities, requesting permission to send a "short term mission" to Turkey, the FAO expressed interest in collaborating with member countries "in order to understand the role of wild birds in H5N1 HPAI and their interactions with domestic poultry."[13] It also emphasised that

[11] Van den Ende, Rinus and Ragip Bayraktar 2008 Sazkoy: 11; Ivanov, Yanko and Ragip Bayraktat 2008 Yorukler: 13

[12] Van den Ende, Rinus and Ragip Bayraktar 2008 Sazkoy: 12; Ivanov, Yanko and Ragip Bayraktat 2008 Yorukler: 15

[13] This correspondence can be found among the attachments of the report from the Joint Mis-

"sampling has not, so far, been targeted around recent confirmed outbreaks in domestic poultry". This shows how Yörükler and other outbreak places turned into strategic places for experts aiming to study the relations between outbreaks among domestic poultry and wild birds; these places thus enact real scale laboratories, and it was just here that *the* buzzard was found.

The buzzard was, according to the report, one out of a total of 39 dead wild birds and two cats that were found and sampled as part of the mission.[14] Moreover, 4 pochards shot dead by hunters had been submitted to the team. Additionally, 177 wild birds of 16 identified species were caught alive and sampled.[15] What made this bird, *the* buzzard, "significant" was that samples taken from this bird and sent to the internationally recognized FAO-OIE reference laboratory in Padova, Italy, tested positive on HPAI H5N1; this was the *only* wild bird that tested positive in this mission, which sought to find a relation between wild birds and HPAI in domestic poultry. In line with Latour, I will argue that this positive laboratory test turned the buzzard into a significant finding while simultaneously making it an immutable mobile, as the positive test result enabled the bird to move and work as "significant" in relation to avian influenza also at distant places. I will return to this point shortly. For now, I will emphasise how, in the FAO-EU joint mission report, the role of this finding, the bird, was uncertain; most likely the buzzard was a victim of its infected prey, but had that been another wild bird or domestic poultry? Moreover, when did the bird become infected with the flu virus? As it is being inscribed in the Joint Mission report, the buzzard carries both the virus *and* the open questions surrounding it.

## Ordering a topology of bioinsecurity

Outbreak places have been strategic sites for studying what I suggest to address as bio*in*security. Sites receive their status as outbreak places on account of the virus entering the area; viruses have found their way *into* these places, thus biosecurity has been violated, borderlines have been transgressed, and life has become *in*secure. I argue that both *in*security and security ought to be addressed, as it is more often than not the former, *in*security, that biosecurity is about; my analysis has shown how biosecurity is about risks and threats towards biosecurity and how this implies that biosecurity in itself tends to be

sion (Newman, Scott Nick Honhold, Javier Sanz-Alvarez and Kiraz Erciyas 2008: 21/ Appendix1).

14 Newman, Scott, Nick Honhold, Javier Sanz-Alvarez and Kiraz Erciyas 2008: Appendix 6

15 Newman, Scott, Nick Honhold, Javier Sanz-Alvarez and Kiraz Erciyas 2008: Appendix 7

taken for granted. Therefore, I argue for a symmetrical attention to matters of both bio*in*security and biosecurity.[16]

The attention that particular outbreak places in Turkey received from international FAO and EU experts was closely related to how outbreak investigations had already contributed to enacting one particular *topology of bioinsecurity* – rather than others. I have analysed outbreak investigation reports in order to study how outbreak places have been enacted as sites of bio*in*security. In Chapter 3, my analysis of the first reported outbreak of HPAI H5N1 virus in Turkey primarily highlights the relevance of bio*in*security as a companion to biosecurity. While my study of this Manyas-outbreak also demonstrates how an outbreak investigation report contributed to enacting one particular topology of bioinsecurity, Chapter 6 offers a far more thorough analysis of this ordering process.

In this latter chapter, I oscillate between outbreak places *out there* in "traditional sense" and the text and illustrations *in* the outbreak investigation reports. I engage what I call three tools for ordering: textualization of space, mapping and the copy/paste tool. My analyses show how these tools contribute to ordering the outbreak places. More specifically, I trace how migratory flyways, particular versions of wetlands inhabited by wild birds, and the practice of backyard poultry have been inscribed in the reports through the use of these tools for ordering. Moreover, I show how this is undertaken in a way that enacts outbreak places as isolated villages and wild bird habitats. The only infrastructure, or way for viruses to enter, inscribed in the outbreak investigation reports is migratory flyways. Hence, the outbreak investigation reports are enacting a context where wild birds become the only possible means for infection.

## Opening up the avian influenza multiple

By oscillating between different sites of inquiry, or by studying the relational space within and between various reports and my own field notes, I have not only seen how outbreak places are being enacted, but also how they might have been enacted differently. This has made it possible to realize how ordering is also about exclusions, and how it involves making particular matters absent and others present. Furthermore, this has enabled me to realize how the topology of bio*in*security enacted in outbreak investigation reports involves efforts for keeping things apart, how it involves separation, and what I have addressed as disarticulating alternatives.[17]

[16] This argument is further developed in Chapter 3

[17] Moser, Ingunn 2008

When the sentence ensuring that "[d]espite extensive inquiry, no evidence could be found for introduction of the virus by movements of animals or people or trade in live poultry or poultry products, or by gifts of the same" was passed on through, and put to work in, several outbreak investigation reports, this did not only have the effect to re-assuring the reader that inquiries had not succeeded in identifying any such source of virus introduction. It also achieved much more; my analysis has shown how this sentence, and the way it is copied and passed on to new documents, also contributes to making the mentioned matters, "animals or people or ( . . . ) live poultry or poultry products, or ( . . . ) gifts of the same", absent.

It was my own observations when visiting the field "out there" that made me aware of this absence *in* the texts; during my visits to outbreak places, which I had learned about through reading outbreak investigation reports, I was struck by the presence of integrated farms well within the 3-kilomtre protection zone. The textualized absence became present in the encounter between outbreak investigation reports and fieldwork observations. Consulting additional reports, which enact poultry as an economic resource, has provided ground from which avian influenza at these outbreak places may just as well be enacted as other versions of a poultry issue; layers are added on the same ground making avian influenza a commercial poultry issue, rather than exclusively a backyard poultry issue; and as a market and trade issue, involving humanly induced mechanisms for spread, rather than exclusively wild birds. In this way, by moving between textual analysis of outbreak investigation reports and my own fieldwork observations, I realized how avian influenza could be enacted in multiple and heterogeneous ways at these particular outbreak places; this is similar to how my detailed analyses of both the Global Strategy and the Turkish National Strategy contributes to *realizing* how avian influenza is enacted as heterogeneous and multiple issues in those documents. In the context of the Turkish outbreak places, there were matters present that could have contributed to enacting avian influenza as an economic issue, as a commercial poultry issue, and as an issue of emergence – all in heterogeneous ways.

## Dealing with frictions: A process of making inner heat productive

Learning how close the industrial poultry farms were located to the backyard poultry places, which were used to forcefully enact avian influenza as a wild bird issue, and observing the absence of alternatives such as just these poultry farms in the outbreak investigation reports, caused a kind of friction that has taken me quite some effort to turn into something more productive than facile conspiracy theories.

It is easy to become caught up in the most obvious answers to the *why*-question: commercial poultry houses were made absent in order to protect the poultry industry, which is considered a locomotive for agricultural development and economic growth. Making this "locomotive" absent when enacting outbreak places in the investigation reports resembles how the so-called "livestock revolution" was not enacted as a threat but rather turned into a victim when avian influenza was enacted as an economic issue in body text of the Global Strategy. Only in the appendix – in the *back matter* of the Global Strategy – was the "livestock revolution" also enacted as a possible cause for the emergence of avian influenza and other transboundary and possibly zoonotic animal diseases.[18] Moreover, given that the Turkish National Strategy states that an estimated 40% of the total poultry production is represented by informal backyard poultry hold, it would be reasonable to conclude that it is a shared interest of the commercial poultry sector and the government to minimise backyard poultry.[19] This would both increase the market for commercial poultry products and expand one important source for state taxation. A third answer to why the commercial sector has been made absent, may relate to the authorities' interest in "cleaning up" practices regarded as primitive, old fashioned, or otherwise unwanted in modern Turkey.[20] A fourth answer can be found within the context of the AI project and the international expert team, who repeatedly expressed great interest in determining the role of wild birds in the outbreaks.[21] This interest fits well with how wild birds entered the final version of the Global Strategy, as analysed in Chapter 5 of this book.

However, my analyses have shown that conspiring interests cannot explain this. Interests are indeed neither clear-cut nor fixed, but rather complex and ever changing. Carrying out fieldwork at outbreak places and interviewing those in charge of outbreak investigations has shown how – despite their absence from the outbreak investigation reports – the poultry houses were indeed taken care of. They were checked for virus contamination both clinically and

---

[18] Please refer to my analysis in Chapters 4 and 6.

[19] Ivanov, Yanko 2007. This is discussed in Chapters 1 and 4 of this volume.

[20] Please refer to Steve Hinchliffe and Nick Bingham (2008b) for a similar concern in relation to Egypt, and to Natalie Porter (2014) in regards to Viet Nam

[21] Interview with international field epidemiologist (referred to in Chapter 1) working for the AI project, *Ankara 29.05.2007* (Interview conducted in English). Other examples where this interest is exemplified is through the delivery of the wild bird catching technique courses and the strong focus on wild birds, wetlands and bird hunters in the outbreak investigation reports

pathologically; moreover, the active surveillance of this poultry was intensified and they were slaughtered prior to the locally standard of 45 days of growth, which is here defined as the optimal age for slaughter.[22]

What can be drawn from this? Or, *how* can we draw something from this that is more productive than facile conspiracy theories? The approach I have chosen has been to just attend to the *how*-question – rather than asking *why*: *How* does this way of ordering outbreak places work? I have argued that the outbreak investigation reports contribute to ordering the complex situation of *outbreak emergencies* in ways that make them governable; the way outbreaks are being ordered in the reports contribute to reducing complexity, hence legitimising disease eradication measures at outbreak places. By not including commercial poultry farms, the controversial measures of culling could be limited to small but uncontrollable free range flocks, while, for example, the batch of approximately 15 000 broilers at Muhtar's poultry house were saved. Furthermore, the outbreak investigation reports contributed to enacting a particular version of the bio*in*secure topology of outbreak places in a way that enabled the epidemiologists to meet the expectations of providing conclusions in regards to the source of infection. Conclusions could be established – not on evidentiary facts, but on a lack of identified alternative sources of infection.

Studying how the ordering of outbreak places involves inclusion and exclusion called into attention processes and effects of *separation*. *Separation* adds to the analytical concepts of inclusion and exclusion by drawing attention to how some versions or matters are made mobile and others not.[23] While various matters related to the commercial poultry sector were handled domestically, for example, as part of the AI project's more general tasks as discussed in Chapters 2 and 6, the outbreak investigation reports contributed to making other matters mobile, thereby enabling these matters to travel, in the form of texts, to the offices of the OIE, the FAO and the WHO.

Hence, these mobile matters, contrary to those matters that remained and were handled domestically, contributed to meeting the demand for knowledge regarding *emergent matters of concern* related to avian influenza spread, and in this way contributed to re-enacting the "global threat" of avian influenza. A vital outcome of my analysis in Chapter 6 was that versions of avian influenza enacted through an *emergency,* as inscribed in the outbreak investigation reports, contributed to meeting the need for knowledge on *emergent* matters of concern. In this regard, this study addresses some implications related to

---

22 Please refer to Chapter 6 for a more detailed account of this matter.

23 Asdal, Kristin 2007

complexity. I have pointed out how making emergencies governable involves reducing complexity. However, filling the emergent need to prepare for unforeseen events, such as disease outbreaks, is likely achieved more efficiently when complexities are taken into account.[24]

## Making "backyard poultry" bioinsecure through separation and generalization

By studying the means through which avian influenza is enacted in Turkey, I have traced how the outbreaks have been explained by virus transmission *from* wild birds *to* backyard poultry. This version of avian influenza as a wild bird- and backyard poultry issue, where wild birds enact the major matter of bio*in*security, goes well together with, and is thus strengthened by, the way Asian smallholder practices or backyard poultry hold have been enacted in the Global Strategy. My analyses have shown how particular poultry farming practices in Asia, as they have been inscribed in the Global Strategy, have been re-inscribed into the Turkish National Strategy.[25] These analyses have shown how vital epidemiological specificities related to farming practices are left behind when the term "backyard poultry" moves to, and continues working within, the National Strategy. I have showed how details commonly regarded as epidemiologically relevant, such as the poultry species involved, density of birds and mobility, are separated from the concept of "backyard poultry". The free ranging nature of the poultry, on the other hand, makes this concept mobile. Characterised as "backyard poultry", flocks of 6 to 60 chicken and hens scavenging in Turkish gardens, come to be as bio*in*secure as large flocks of ducks, kept on rice fields and moved across regions in Asia; by applying the general term "backyard poultry" this heterogeneous farming practice come to be enacted as bio*in*secure across distance and despite difference.

## Separating matters of fact and matters of concern, and excluding the option of environmental pollution

The way viral flow is being enacted – as unidirectional, from wild to domestic – has been a recurring matter of concern throughout this book. Detailed analyses have shown how other modes of ordering the topology of outbreak places could

[24] Hinchliffe, Steve 2001; Hinchliffe, Steve 2013; Hinchliffe, Steve, John Allen, Stephanie Lavau, Nick Bingham and Simon Carter2012; Hinchliffe, Steve and Stephanie Lavau 2013. For a similar point on farming practices and a more general discussion about complexities, please refer to Singleton, Vicky 2010.

[25] Please refer to Chapter 4 for a detailed analysis of this issue

just as well have enabled viral flow in the opposite direction, from domestic to wild. In this way, I have highlighted how avian influenza both in Turkey and "globally" as enacted in the Global Strategy, could just as well have been enacted as an environmental issue. When that is not happening, it can be seen in relation to how emergence, in the sense of virus turning from low- to high pathogenic, is not a matter of concern.

As my analysis of the strategy documents in Chapter 4 shows, it is taken as a matter of fact that this crucial genetic change is enabled by certain conditions that are present within intensive poultry farming practices. While wild birds may introduce low pathogenic avian influenza virus to domestic birds, it is within and among poultry living under these farming conditions that the virus supposedly may turn highly pathogenic. As my analysis shows, these facts remain in the appendix, in the back matter, of the Global Strategy. The matter of concern enacted in the body text of the Global Strategy is an already existing highly pathogenic avian influenza virus. This appears to be the case in Turkey too. When studying avian influenza in Turkey at multiple sites, avian influenza outbreaks is about spread *into* the country or farm from an external location, from the outside. Spread in the other direction, from domestic to wild, becomes a concern in relation to other agricultural/hydrological issues that are handled separately from avian influenza. This became apparent as I included water quality studies in order to re-enact the topology of outbreak places, in Chapter 6.

As an interesting contrast to the outbreak investigation reports carried out by the AI project, which provided "strong evidence" of a wild bird source of infection of the backyard poultry flocks infected as part of the Black Sea outbreaks, the joint mission report did not formulate such strong statements with regard to the infected buzzard. Also, while the FAO-EU joint mission report enacted wild birds as the most likely means for introduction, it did provide space for uncertainty regarding the source of infection:

> Based on the foraging behaviour of the buzzard, infection most likely took place by ingestion of a sick live (moribund) or fresh dead bird carcass, with the greatest likelihood being a dead wild bird since infected poultry had been culled 3–4 weeks prior to this bird becoming infected. There is also a possibility that the buzzard was infected a few weeks prior, when there were both infected wild and domestic poultry, but only succumbed much later.[26]

As we can see in this text, despite uncertainty, one option – that other wild birds were the source of infection – is enacted as the "greatest likelihood". The

[26] Newman, Scott Nick Honhold, Javier Sanz-Alvarez and Kiraz Erciyas 2008:15

other less likely "possibility" is that the buzzard has been infected for a while, and therefore both a wild and domestic source would be possible. While the report separates between less likely and more likely sources of infection, it does, importantly, enact uncertainty by including both options.

## Mobile and immobile matters of concern

I will emphasise the point, in regard to the relation between separation and mobility and some vital effects thereof, by bringing in a particular official letter. As the title says, this is the letter of "Declaration of Freedom from Notifiable Avian Influenza". It is referring to the so-called Black Sea outbreaks, and was sent by Assoc. Prof. Dr. Muzaffer Aydemir, General Director of MARA's General Directorate of Protection and Control, to Dr. Bernard Vallat, Director General of the OIE in Paris, on July 14, 2008.[27]

Included with the declaration letter is the Final Report on Outbreaks Eradication and Post-Outbreak Surveillance. This final report consists of nine pages where the "source of outbreak" is "determined"; By referring to the outbreak investigations, the reports of which are analysed in Chapter 6, MARA states that the "source of outbreak has been determined as direct or indirect contact with wild birds."[28] The report continues: "There has been contact with infectious materials (feathers and viscera) from hunted wild birds or hunting cartridges in the indirect contact cases." Again, this is based on the conclusions drawn from the outbreak investigation of each single case explored in Chapter 6 of this book. My analyses of the individual reports show that in all of the cases, "infectious materials" were not available for examination at the time of investigation. It was either consumed – hunted birds by the hunter and his family, and the remnants by the backyard poultry – or it had in other ways been lost before the outbreaks were investigated.[29]

In this context, ornithological observations and the textualization of space played a crucial role in the ordering of the outbreak event. A closer examination of MARA's final report attached to the letter of declaration of freedom from disease brings to light how ornithological observations contributed to bringing the investigations closer to the source of the outbreak:

> Census work at these sites demonstrated that many bridge species (birds that move between backyard households where domestic birds are kept, and wild birds habitat)

[27] Aydemir, Muzaffer 2008

[28] Ibid., note, the words are underlined in the original text.

[29] Van den Ende, Rinus and Ragip Bayraktar 2008 Sazkoy

could have come into direct contact with infectious materials discarded from hunted birds, or directly contact with infected poultry.[30]

It is as an extension to this that *the* buzzard re-enters the scene. The letter from MARA continues: "A buzzard (buteo buteo), found moribund and euthanized, near the Yörükler site on 5 March 2008 was positive for H5N1-HPAI based on diagnostics at the Padova FAO-OIE Reference Laboratory."[31] The characteristics it brings along to Paris is that it was found near one of the outbreak places in the liminal state between life and death, and that it, according to internationally recognised laboratory tests, was a carrier of the HPAI H5N1 virus. However, left behind and not brought along to Paris are all the uncertainties regarding what relation the buzzard had to the outbreak; these uncertainties and open questions were surrounding this "significant finding" as it was first inscribed in the FAO-EU joint mission report. The buzzard is now working as a *mutable mobile*; it is bringing some characteristics along, such as the fact that is was involved in the outbreaks, while others, specifically the uncertainties and concerns related to how it was involved, are left behind.[32]

## Enacting the global: The dead buzzard arrives, fit and famous, at the centre of global governance

After setting off from the Black Sea wetlands and travelling via Ankara, the buzzard arrived in Paris. There, in Paris, the quality of being found HPAI positive nearby an outbreak place brings the buzzard on the stage for a third time: Its story from the avian flu infected wetlands is broadcasted worldwide in the three official OIE languages – English, French and Spanish – via the quarterly *OIE Bulletin*. Here the whole story, as it is told in the final report of MARA, is published.[33]

This issue of the *Bulletin* is devoted to *Wildlife*. Under the heading "Improving wildlife surveillance for its protection while protecting us from the disease it transmits", Vallat, the Director General of the OIE, emphasises the threat of "wildlife diseases".[34] His editorial opens by making the following an undisputable fact: "Wildlife diseases are a growing concern worldwide. In addition to threatening populations of wild animals themselves, *wildlife disease can affect domestic animals and human health*." The last part, which I

30 Aydemir, Muzaffer 2008

31 Aydemir, Muzaffer 2008

32 For more on this issue, please refer to Chapter 4 where I discuss the various ways in which "backyard poultry" moved from Asia, via the Global Strategy, to Turkey. See also above.

33 OIE 2008: 38–43

34 OIE 2008: 1

stress by setting it in italics, stands out as a highlighted quotation and catches the reader's eye; it clearly and explicitly states the major matters of concern: Avian influenza does not represent a *poultry disease.*[35] Rather, it is classified as one of many threatening "[w]ildlife diseases [that] can affect domestic animals and human health".

Following this buzzard demonstrates how *the global avian influenza concern,* what the Global Strategy and Turkish National Strategy refer to as "the global crisis" and what Vallat here characterizes as "the avian influenza global crisis", is not pre-given but rather something that is *becoming* through processes and relations; through inclusions and exclusions, by simultaneous making of presence and absence, or what Law and Mol call "conjoint alterity".[36] The "global" avian influenza issue is being enacted within what Law and Mol suggest to see as the topological structures of fire space. What I have done through my analysis presented in this book (and partially extended in this chapter), is to address some of these processes and relations; I have been moving with(in) and following some of the "earthly relations" through which avian influenza is being enacted; I have studied how avian influenza is being textualized and inscribed, I have analysed these "flickering star patterns"[37] and "global connections"[38] through which avian influenza is being ordered.

In doing so, I have also showed how "the global" *is* local – and not only made up by the local. I have suggested the notion of *connecting locals* in order to study what is commonly referred to as global-local relations. This implies a horizontal approach; rather than seeing the global-local as a vertical top/bottom, or above/grass-root relation, where influences and movement travel in one direction or the other, and where "the global" may be locally adjusted, adapted or simply taken up unchanged, the notion of connecting locals works to emphasise the relational and processual nature of local and global issues alike; the notion *connecting locals* invites for studying how both "the local" and "the global" are the current outcome of on-going processes and relations; it emphasises how places – like any form of reality – are not static and pre-given but changing.

For example, Kızıksa village, which I introduced on Chapters 2 and 3, and Yörükler where *the* buzzard was found, turned into outbreak places as certain relations were made – rather others. Chapter 6 further highlights this; for

---

35 OIE Terrestrial Animal Health Code Chapter 10.4. Avian influenza http://www.oie.int/eng/normes/mcode/en_chapitre_1.10.4.pdf, accessed on 20.08.2014

36 Law, John and Annemarie Mol 2001: 620

37 Law, John and Annemarie Mol 2001

38 Tsing, Anna 2005

example, if other geographical features and other relations were inscribed in the report on the Yörükler outbreak place, this wetland area could have been enacted in a different way. As a result, this area would not necessarily have been enacted as exclusively a wild bird habitat and source of infection from outside; it could have been enacted as an area with agricultural runoff water and domestic pollution. Hence, avian influenza would have become an environmental issue where wildlife would be subject to infection *from* commercial farms. The FAO-EU joint mission report did indeed open for this. As my analysis above shows, the report conveys uncertainty in regard to the role of *the* infected buzzard. In this case though, these uncertainties were matters of concern that did *not* move along with the bird. As a matter of fact, stabilized by positive test results from a recognised laboratory, the bird was infected with the HPAI H5N1 virus, and it was this *diagnosed version of the bird* that was made mobile and which contributed to enacting what Vallat refers to as *the worldwide concern of wildlife diseases*. This highlights how the local may be seen, like Law has suggested, as ponds in ponds and the various versions move, co-exist, connect and influence each other in different ways.[39]

An overall ambition has been to contribute to interference; to contribute to enacting something different rather than re-enforcing already established versions of avian influenza as *a* "global concern".[40] Bringing in this particular buzzard in this final chapter is not done in order to contribute to its fame. Rather, I use this bird as a tool for interference by addressing how it obtained its role and how it came to enact avian influenza as a worldwide wildlife concern in the way it does – rather than other ways: When re-enacting avian influenza as a wild bird issue, I have done this by showing how this is one (heterogeneous) version, but that there are also other ways in which avian influenza could have been enacted as a wild life issue; that wild birds are being enacted as *threatening* is not pre-given. Rather, what my analysis has shown is how this was the outcome of processes and relations; the way OIE and Vallat contribute to enacting avian influenza and other transboundary diseases as wildlife diseases is the outcome of connecting locals, I argue; it was the outcome of certain versions of the event, rather than other possible versions. That is, in the words of Law and Mol, conjoined alterities. By attending to the specificities, to the local

[39] On Law's use of Leibnitz' metaphor of a pond in a pond, please refer to Chapters 1 and for discussion and references.

[40] Ingunn Moser's (2008) account on "Making Alzheimer's disease matter" should here, again, be acknowledged as one of the strongest sources of influence. Please also refer to my discussion on feminist technoscience in Chapter 1. For a classical contribution see e.g. Haraway, Donna 1997

formation of issues, and to the way they travel (or not) and go together (or not) with other issues and versions thereof, this work has contributed to *realizing* for example how wild birds – which are enacted as matters of bio*in*security and a threat – could just as well have been enacted as *threatened*. This is important because it highlights how bio-matters come to matter – and how they come to matter as global concerns, calling for particular interventions – rather than others.

## Re-thinking the effects of exclusion

Making the commercial sector absent, through exclusion and lack of inclusion, has enabled wild birds to be enacted as threatening and backyard poultry hold as bio*in*secure. In addition, my analyses have shown how the absence of the commercial poultry sector in outbreak investigation reports has had an empowering effect on certain parts of this heterogeneous sector. Attending to the excluded, in a manner advocated by feminist scholars of STS, my study has also shown how the relation between exclusion and marginalization should not be taken for granted. In the case of avian influenza in Turkey, I have argued that by being excluded when the topology of outbreak places is enacted, the commercial poultry sector has remained "clean"; by not being part of the topology of bio*in*security, this sector has managed to remain biosecure. Again, attending to specificities and internal variation, which is another analytical concern stressed by feminist STS scholars, this study has also addressed how the commercial poultry sector is heterogeneous; accordingly, there are variations within the commercial poultry sector with regard to how various firms survived the avian influenza crisis (or not).

Arriving the end of this study on the becoming of avian influenza in the space between Turkish outbreak places and textual sites of the global governance of disease, it is striking to realize something that did not cross my way: despite the generally accepted fact that HPAI emerges within systems of intensive poultry production, and even though the assumption that emerging transboundary animal diseases will be more common in the future due to increased consumer demands leading to intensified production and accelerating worldwide transportation of poultry products, it does not appear to be an option for HPAI control to suggest alternative non-animal sources of protein. That this alternative is *not* articulated as part of disease control highlights how governing avian influenza is just as much about securing the poultry industry as it is about controlling disease.

# References

Agrawal, Arun 2005: *Environmentality: Technologies of Government and the Making of Subjects*, Duke University Press: Durham

AI project 2007: *Epidemiology, Training and Local Experts Field Visit, Risk Assessment and Biosecurity Improvement in Backyard Poultry Farms*, Unpublished Mission Report, Technical Assistance to Avian Influenza Preparedness and Response Project, Turkey. Ankara

AI project 2008: *An Overview of Wild Bird Mediated High Pathogenic H5N1 Avian Influenza in Turkey, 2005 – 2008*. Report the webpage of the Technical Assistance to Avian Influenza Preparedness and Response Project, Turkey. http://www.prwatson.co.uk/TR_06_AI_SV/English/Reports/Wild %20bird%20mediated%20H5N1%20HPAI%20Turkey.pdf, (accessed on 04.08.2014)

Akbay, C and I. Boz 2005: "Turkey's livestock sector: Production, consumption and policies",*in Livestock Research for Rural Development*, Vol. 17, Issue 9

Akrich, Madeleine 1992: "The De-Scription of Technical Objects", pp. 205–224 in Wiebe E. Bijker and John Law (Eds.): *Shaping Technology, Building Society: Studies in Sociotechnical Change*, Cambridge, Mass: MIT Press

Althusser, Louis 1971: *On Ideology*. New Left Books: London

Altındeğer, Mustafa and Burhan Hekimoğlu 2010: *Samsun'da Kanatlı Eti Sektörü* [Report on Poultry Meat Sector in Samsun]. T.C. Samsun Valiliği,İl Taım Müdürlğü. Samsu

Aral Y, Cengis, Yalcin, Yavuz Cevger, Cevat Sipahi, Savaş Sariözkan 2010: "Financial effects of the highly pathogenic avian influenza outbreaks on the Turkish broiler producers", in *Poultry Science*, Vol. 89, Issue 5, pp. 1085–1088

Arik, Musa, Yanki Ivanov, Ragip Bayraktar, Marinus Van den Ende 2007: *Avian Influenza Surveillance Manual*.Technical Assistance to Avian Influenza Preparedness and Response Project, Turkey. http://www.prwatson.co.uk/TR_06_AI_SV/English/Reports/AI%20S urveillance%20Manual.pdf, (accessedon 04.08.2014)

Asdal, Kristin 2005: *Grensetrafikk. Nedslag i veterinærvesenets historie*. Unipub Forlag: Oslo

Asdal, Kristin 2007: "Re-Inventing Politics of the State. Science and the Politics of Contestation" in Kristin Asdal, Brita Brenna and Ingunn Moser (Eds.) 2007: *Technoscience. The Politics of Interventions*, Unipub: Oslo

Asdal, Kristin 2008a: Enacting things through numbers: Taking nature into account/ing, Geoforum No. 39, pp. 123–132

Asdal, Kristin 2008b: "On Politics and the little Tools of Democracy: A Down to Earth Approach", *Distinction* No. 16, pp. 11–26 (16p)

Asdal, Kristin 2008c: "Subjected to Parliament: The Laboratory of Experimental Medicine and the Animal Body", Social Studies of Science Vol. 38, Issue 6: 89–91

Asdal, Kristin 2011a: *Politikkens natur – Naturens politikk*, Universitetsforlaget, Oslo

Asdal, Kristin 2011b: "The Office: The Weakness of Numbers and the Production of Non-Authority." *Accounting, Organizations and Society* Vol. 36, Issue 1, pp. 1–9

Asdal, Kristin 2012: "Contexts in Actions – and the Future of the Past in STS", in *Science, Technology and Human Values*, Vol. 37, Issue 4

Asdal, Kristin 2014: "Versions of milk and versions of care: The emergence of mother's milk as an interested object and medicine as a form of dispassionate care", *in Science in Context*, Vol. 27, Special Issue 02, 1850–1980, pp. 307–331

Asdal, Kristin, Anne-Jorunn Berg, Brita Brenna, Ingunn Moser and Linda M. Rustad 1998: *Betatt av viten. Bruksanvisninger til Donna Haraway.* Spartacus Forlag, Oslo

Asdal, Kristin, Kjell Lars Berge, Karen Gammelgaard, Helge Jordheim, Tore Rem, Trygve Riiser-Gundersen og Johan L. Tønnesen 2008: *Tekst og historie. Å lese tekster historisk*. Universitetsforlaget: Oslo

Asdal Kristin, C. Borch and Ingunn Moser 2008: "Editorial: The technologies of politics", *Distinktion: Scandinavian Journal of Social Theory*, Vol. 16, pp. 5–10

Asdal, Kristin, Brita Brenna and Ingunn Moser (Red.) 2001: *Teknovitenskaplige kulturer*. Spartakus Forlag AS

Asdal, Kristin, Brita Brenna and Ingunn Moser (Eds.) 2007: *Technoscience. The Politics of Interventions*, Unipub: Oslo

Asdal, Kristin and Ingunn Moser 2012: "Experiments in Context and Contexting", in *Science, Technology and Human Values*, Vol. 37, Issue 4, pp. 291–206.

Aşkaroğlu, Haluk H., Yanko Ivanov and Ragip Bayraktar 2008: *Manual on Poultry Manure and Carcass Management*. Technical Assistance to Avian Influenza Preparedness and Response Project, Turkey

Austin, John L. 1975: *How to Do Things with Words*. 2nd ed. Cambridge, MA: Harvard University Press

Aydemir, Muzaffer 2008: *Declaration of Freedom from Notifiable Avian Influenza*. Letter attached to Newman, Scott, Nick Honhold, Javier Sanz-Alvarez and Kiraz Erciyas 2008: *Investigation of the role of wild birds in highly pathogenic avian influenza outbreaks in Turkey between January and February 2008*. Mission Report, Food and Agriculture Organization of the United Nations, Crisis Management Centre – Animal Health and Animal Health Division- EMPRES, Rome, Italy.

Bakan, Gülfem, Hülya Böke Özkoç, Sevtap Tülek and Hüseyin Cüce 2010: "Integrated Environmental Quality Assessment of Kıırmak River and its Coastal Environment",*Turkish Journal of Fisheries and Aquatic Sciences* Vol. 10, pp. 453–462

Barad, K., 2003: Posthumanist performativity: toward an understanding of how matter comes to matter, Signs. Journal of Women in Culture and Society 28 (3), pp. 80–83

Barad K 2007: *Meeting the universe halfway: quantum physics and the entanglment of matter and meaning,* Duke University Press, Durham NC

Barker, Kezia 2008: "Flexible boundaries in biosecurity: accommodating gorse in Aotearoa NewZealand", in *Environment and Planning A*, Vol. 40, pp. 1598–1614

Barret, Ron and Peter J. Brown 2008: "Stigma in the Time of Influenza: Social and Institutional Responses to Pandemic Emergencies", in *The Journal of Infectious Diseases* Vol. 197, pp. 34–37

Barry, Andrew 2001: *Political Machines. Governing a Technological Society*. The Athlone Press. London and New York

Bayraktar, Ragıp 2007: "Extension Report Period covered: 01-February-07 to 12-March-07 inclusive." http://www.prwatson.co.uk/TR_06_AI_SV/English/Reports/Extension%20Report%20Feb-Mar%2007.pdf, *accessed on 04.08.2014*

BBC 2007: *Farming Today* This Week, Radio 4, 11 August

Bingham, Nick and Steve Hinchliffe 2008: "Mapping the multiplicities of Biosecurity", in Lakoff, Andrew and Stephen Collier (Eds.): *Biosecurity Interventions*, Columbia University Press: New Yor

Braun, Bruce 2007:"Biopolitics and the molecularization of life", in *Cultural Geographies* Issue 14, Vol. 6

Brenna, Brita 2012: Natures, Contexts, and Natural History" in *Science, Technology and Human Values*, Vol. 37, Issue 4, pp. 355–378

Buller, Henry 2013: "Animal geographies I", in *Progress in Hu-*

*man Geography*, Published online on 21 March 2013, DOI: 10.1177/0309132513479295

Butler, Declan 2006: "Doubts hang over source of bird flu spread", in *Nature*, Vol. 439, Issue 16, February

Callon, Michel 1986: "Some Elements of a Sociology of Translation", in John Law (ed.): *Power Action and Belief. A New Sociology of Knowledge? Sociological Review Monograph* 32. Reprinted in Asdal, Kristin, Brita Brenna and Ingunn Moser (Eds.) 2007: *Technoscience. The Politics of Interventions*, Unipub

Delany, Simon, Jan Veen and Jacquie Clark (Eds.) 2006: *Urgent preliminary assessment of ornithological data relevant to the spread of Avian Influenza in Europe,* Report by EURING and wetlands international to the European Commission, Study contract N°07010401/2005/425926/MAR/B4

Delany, Brouwer and Veen (Eds.) 2007: *Ornithological data relevant to the spread of Avian Influenza in Europe (phase 2). Further identification and first field assessment of Higher Risk Species*, Wetlands International, Wageningen, The Netherlands

Chen et al. 2006: Establishment of multiple sublineages of H5N1 influenza-virus in Asia: Implications for pandemic control", by*PNAS/The National Academy of Sciences of the USA*. Vol. 103, Issue 8, pp. 2845–2850.

Full list of authors: Chen H, Li KS, Wang J, Fan XH, Rayner JM, Vijaykrishna D, Zhang JX,Zhang LJ, Guo CT, Cheung CL, Xu KM, Duan L, Huang K, Qin K,Leung YHC, Wu WL, Lu HR, Chen Y, Xia NS, Naipospos TSP, YuenKY, Hassan SS, Bahri S, Nguyen TD, Webster RG, Peiris JSM and Guan Y.

Deleuze, Gilles 1993: *The Fold: Leibniz and the Baroque*, Athlone Press, London

Didrickson, Özgür Keşaplı, Özge Keşaplı Can and Can Bilgin 2007: *Identifying the Role of Wild Birds as a Vector and Transmitter of Avian Influenza in Turkey (pilot study)*, Report by Kuş Araştirmaları Derneği (KAD), Ankara

Dobson, Andrew, Kezia Barker and Sarah L. Taylor (Eds.) 2013: *Biosecurity: the socio-politics of invasive species and infectious diseases.* Earthscan/ Routledge.

Dolberg, Frands, Emmanuelle Guerne Bleich and Anni McLeod 2005: Emergency Regional Support for Post-Avian Influenza Rehabilitation TCP/RAS/3010(E), Summary of projects and outcome, Food and Agriculture Organization of the United Nations, http://www.fao.org/docs /eims/upload/211941/poultrysector_seasiasummary_en.pdf (accessed on 20.08.2014)

Donaldson, Andrew and David Wood 2004: "Surveilling Strange Materialities: Categorisation in the Evolving Geographies of FMD biosecurity",in *Environment and Planning D: Society and Space,* Vol. 22, pp. 373–391

Dorwart, Reinhold A. 1959: "Cattle Disease (Rinderpest?) – Prevention and Cure in Brandenburg, 1665–1732", in *Agricultural history,* University of California Press

Downey, Gary Lee, Joseph Dumit and Sharon Traweek (Eds.) 1995: "Cyborgs and Citadels: Anthropological Interventions in Emerging Sciences and Technologies." in*Emerging Sciences and Technologie*s. Santa Fe, NM: School Am. Res. Pres

Durutan, Nedret and Okan, Cüneyt n.d.: *Turkey Poultry Biosecurity Presentation. Backyard and Small Scale Commercial Production.* Presentation, World Bank. Ankara

Durutan, Nedret and Okan, Cüneyt 2006: *An Assessment of Avian Influenza Impacts in Backyard Poultry in Turke*y, World Bank, Ankar

EFSA 13/09/2005: *Animal health and welfare aspects of Avian Influenza* Scientific, report 126 pages, Annex to The EFSA 2005: Journa*l Animal health and welfare aspects of Avian Influenza* 266, pp. –21 (Opinion of the Scientific Panel on Animal Health and Welfare (AHAW) on a request from the Commission related to animal health and welfare aspects of Avian Influenza Question number: EFSA-Q-2004–075, Adopted13/09/2005

EFSA 12/05/2006: *Opinion of the Scientific Panel Animal Health and Welfare(AHAW) related with the Migratory Birds and their Possible Role in the Spread of Highly Pathogenic Avian Influenza* Question number: EFSAQ-2005–243, Adopted 12/05/200

Emerson, Robert, Rachel Fretz and Linda Shaw 1995: *Writing Ethnographic Field Notes.* University of Chicago Press: Chicago

Enticott, Gareth 2008:"The spaces of biosecurity: prescribing and negotiating solutions to bovine tuberculosis", in *Environment and Planning A*, Vol. 40, pp. 1568–1582

Fangen, Katrine 2005: "Deltagande observations", pp. 117 – 134. Liber förlag. Stockholm

FAO 2001 March: *Biosecurity in Food and Agriculture,* FAO Committee on Agriculture, 16th session, Rome 26–30 March. As of 20.08.2014 available on http://www.fao.org/docrep/MEETING/003/X9181e.HTM

FAO 2003 April: *Biosecurity in Food and Agriculture,* FAO Committee on Agriculture 17th session, Rome 31. March – 4. April. As of 20.08.2014 available on: http://www.fao.org/docrep/MEETING/006/Y8453E.HTM

FAO 2004 Sept.: *FAO Recommendations on the Prevention, Control and*

*Eradication of Highly Pathogenic Avian Influenza (HPAI) in Asia (proposed with the support of the OIE).* Position paper of the Food and Agriculture Organization of the United Nations. As of 20.08.2014 available on: http://web.oie.int/eng/AVIAN_INFLUENZA/FAO%20recommendations%20on%20HPAI.pdf

FAO 2007: *FAO Biosecurity Tool Kit*, Food and Agriculture Organization of the United Nations: Rome. As of 20.08.2014 available on: ftp://ftp.fao.org/docrep/fao/010/a1140e/a1140e.pdf

FAO 2008: *Biosecurity for highly pathogenic avian influenza. Issues and options.* FAO Animal Production and Health Paper. Food and Agricultural Organization of the United Nation. Rome. ISSN 0254–6019. As of 20.08.2014 available on: ftp://ftp.fao.org/docrep/fao/011/i0359e/i0359e00.pdf

FAO/ECTAD 2006: *Highly Pathogenic Avian Influenza in Africa A Strategy and Proposed Programme to Limit Spread and Build Capacity for Epizootic Disease Control*, Food and Agriculture Organization of the United Nation, Emergency Centre for Transboundary Animal Disease ECTA

FAO/ECTAD 2008 Nov: *Avian Flu: FAO in Action.* Newsletter Number 12. Food and Agriculture Organization of the United Nation, Emergency Centre for Transboundary Animal Diseases. As of 20.08.2014 available on: ftp://ftp.fao.org/docrep/fao/011/aj210e/aj210e00.pdf

FAO and OIE 2004 May: *The Global Framework for the Progressive Control of Transboundary Animal Diseases (GF-TADs)*, Food and Agriculture Organization of the United Nations and World Organisation for Animal Health (OIE). Rome and Paris. As of 20.08.2014 available on: http://www.oie.int/fileadmin/Home/eng/About_us/docs/pdf/GF-TADs_approved_version24May2004.pdf

FAO and OIE 2007 March: *The Global Strategy for Prevention and Control of H5N1 Highly Pathogenic Avian Influenza.* Food and Agriculture Organization and the World Organisation for Animal Health in collaboration with the World Health Organization. As of 20.08.2014 available on: http://www.fao.org/docrep/010/a1145e/a1145e00.htm

FAO, OIE and WHO 2004: *Report of the WHO/FAO/OIE joint consultation on emerging zoonotic diseases*.Food and Agriculture Organization of the United Nations (FAO), World Health Organization (WHO), and World Organisation for Animal Health (OIE).in collaboration with the Health Council of the Netherlands, (HO/CDS/CPE/ZFK/2004.9) 3.–5. May, Geneva, Switzerland. As of 20.08.2014 available on: http://whqlibdoc.who.int/hq/2004/who_cds_cpe_zfk_2004.9.pdf

FAO, OIE and WHO 2005 May [Draft version]: *A Global Strategy for the Progressive Control of Highly Pathogenic Avian Influenza (HPAI)*, Food and Agriculture Organization (FAO, Rome), World Organisation for Animal Health (OIE, Paris) in collaboration with the World Health Organization (WHO, Geneva)

FAO, OIE and WHO 2005 Nov [Final version]: *A Global Strategy for the Progressive Control of Highly Pathogenic Avian Influenza (HPAI)*, Food and Agriculture Organization (FAO, Rome), World Organisation for Animal Health (OIE, Paris) in collaboration with the World Health Organization (WHO, Geneva), As of 20.08.2014 available on: http://www.oie.int/doc/ged/D2891.PDF

FAO, OIE, UNSIC, Unicef, WB and WHO 2008: *Contributing to One World, One Health* A Strategic Framework for Reducing Risks of Infectious Diseases at the Animal–Huma–Ecosystems Interface*, consultation document, October 1$^{4t}$h. Food and Agriculture Organization of the United Nation, the World Organization for Animal Health, United Nations System Influenza Coordination, Unicef and The World Bank and World Health Organization. As of 20.08.2014 available on: http://www.fao.org/docrep/011/aj137e/aj137e00.HTM

Fear, C. J. 2006: "Fish farming and the risk of spread of avian influenza" report on Wild Wings Bird Management and Birdlife International,http://www.birdlife.org/action/science/species/avian_flu/index.html, As of 20.08.2014 available on: http://naturecanada.ca/pdf/BLI_fish_farming_review.pdf,

Fear, Chris J. and Maï Yasué 2006: "Asymptomatic infection with highly pathogenic avian influenza H5N1 in wild birds: how sound is the evidence?*Virology Journal*, Vol. 3, Issue 96

Featherstone David and Joe Painter (Eds.) 2013: *Spatial Politics. Essays for Doreen Massey*. Wiley-Blackwell

Foucault, Michel 2003: *Society must be defended: Lectures at the Collège de France 1975–197.6* Allen Lane

Foucault, Michel 2007: *Security, Territory, Population: Lectures at the College de France 1977–1978*. New York: Palgrave Macmillan.

Foucault, Michel 2010: *The Birth of Biopolitics: Lectures at the Collège de France, 1978–1979*, Palgrave Macmillan

Fox, Patrick 1989: "From Senility to Alzheimer's disease: the rise of the Alzheimer's disease movement."*The Milbank Quarterly* Vol. 67, Issue 1, pp. 5–10

Geerlings, Ellen 2006: *Rapid assessment of HPAI Socio-economic impacts in Turkey*. Food and Agriculture Organization of the United Nations/AGAL

Gilbert, Marius, Xiangming Xiao, Joseph Domenech, Juan Lubroth, Vincent Martin and Jan Slingenbergh 2006: "Anatidae Migration in the Western Palearctic and Spread of Highly Pathogenic Avian Influenza H5N1 Virus", in *EmergingInfectious Diseases* Vol. 12, No. 11, November

Government of Turkey Dec. 2005: *Project Information Document (PID) – Appraisal Stage*, project name "Avian Influenza and Human Pandemic Preparedness and Response", Report No.: AB2025, Undersecretariat of Treasury, Ministry of Agriculture and Rural Affairs and Ministry of Health, Turkey

Greger, Michael 2006: *Bird flu: a virus of our own hatching.* Lantern Books

Habraken, Jolanda M, Jeannette Pols, Patrick JE Bindels and Dick L Willems 2008:"The silence of patients with end-stage COPD:a qualitative study", in*British Journal of General Practice*, Vol. 58 no. 557, pp. 844–849

Hansard, 2001: House of Commons Parliamentary Debates [6t]h Series, Vol. 366, Column 705, Part 69, The Staionery Office, London

Haraway, Donna 1985: "A Manifesto for Cyborgs: Science Technology and Socialist Feminism in the 1980's", in*Socialist Revie*w. Vol. 80, pp. 65–10

Haraway, Donna 1986: "Primatology is Politics by Other Means" in Bleier, Ruth (Ed.) 1986: *Feminist Approaches to Science*, pp. 77–118. Pergamon Press: New York

Haraway, Donna J. 1991: *Simians, Cyborgs, and Women. The Reinvention of Nature*. Routledge: New York

Haraway, Donna J. 1997: *Modest_Witness@Second_Millenium. FemaleMan©_Meets_OncoMouse™. Routledge: London, New York*

Haraway, Donna 2007 [1991]: "Situated Knowledges: The Science Question in Feminism and the Privilege of Partial Perspective" in*Simians, Cyborgs and Women: The Reinvention of Partial Perspective.* Reprinted in Asdal, Kristin, Brita Brenna and Ingunn Moser 2007: *Technoscience. The Politics of Interventions*, Unipub

Haraway, J. Donna 2008: *When Species Meet*. University of Minnesota Press: United States of America

Harding, Sandra 2000: "After the common era", *Journal of Women in Culture and Society*, Vol. 25, no. 4

Harris, Ali S. and Keil, Roger 2007: "Governing the Sick City: Urban Governance in the Age of Emerging Infectious Disease", in*Antipod*, Vol. 9, pp. 846–873

Hecht, Gabrielle 2012: *Being nuclear: Africans and the global uranium trade.* Massachusetts Institute of Technology

Hinchliffe, Steve 2001: "Indeterminacy in-decisions: science, policy and politics in the BSE crisis", in *Transactions of the Institute of British Geographers, New Series* Vol. 26, pp. 182–204

Hinchliffe, Steve 2013: "The insecurity of biosecurity: Re-making emergent infectious diseases", in Dobson, Andrew, Kezia Barker and Sarah L. Taylor (Eds.): *Biosecurity: the socio-politics of invasive species and infectious diseases*. Earthscan/ Routledge

Hinchliffe, Steve, John Allen, Stephanie Lavau, Nick Bingham and Simon Carter 2012: "Biosecurity and the topologies of infected life: from borderlines to borderlands", i*n Transactions of the Institute of British Geographers*. Royal Geographical Society with the Institute of British Geographers

Hinchliffe, Steve and Bingham, Nick 2008a: "People, animals and biosecurity in and through cities" in: Harris, Ali S. and Keil, Roger (Eds.): *Networked Disease: Emerging infections in the global city*. Oxford: U

Hinchliffe, Steve and Nick Bingham 2008b: "Securing life: the emerging practices of biosecurity", in *Environment and Planning A*, Vol. 40, pp. 1534–1551

Hinchliffe, Steve and Stephanie Lavau 2013: "Differentiated circuits: the ecologies of knowing and securing life", in*Environment and Planning D: Society and Space*, Volume 31, pp. 259–274

Hinchliffe, Steve and Sarah Whatmore 2006: Living cities: towards a politics of conviviality", in *Science as Culture*, Vol. 15, Issue 2, pp. 123–13

Honhold, Nick and Ragip Bayraktar 2007 Diyarbakir and Batman: Epidemiology Orinithology Surveys Expert Field Visit, Back to Office Report on Avian Influenza Outbreak in Batman Province", Annex E -"Details of 2007 AI Outbreak in Batman &Diyarbakir" attached to Ivanov, Yanko, Paul, Watson, Rinus Van den Ende and Hélène Vidon: Inception report March EU Project No TR 06.AI/SV Technical Assistance to the Avian Influenza Preparedness and Response. Ankara, Turkey

Ivanov, Yanko 2007: *Strategy for Highly Pathogenic Avian Influenza Preparedness and Control in Turkey*.The European Union's Technical Assistance Programme for Turkey, Technical Assistance to Avian Influenza Preparedness & Response Project, Turke (TR 06.AI/SV), August. Ankara

Ivanov, Yanko and Ragip Bayraktat 2008 Yorukler: *Avian Influenza Outbreak Investigation Mission Report in Yorukler Village/ Samsun province*. Technical Assistance to Avian Influenza Preparedness and Response Project, Turkey. As of 21.08.2014 avaiable on: http://www.prwatson.co.uk/TR_06_AI_SV/English/Reports/Yorukler%20oubreak.pdf

Karafistan, Aysel and Fatma Arik-Colakoglu 2005: "Physical, Chemical and

Microbiological Water Quality of the Manyas Lake, Turkey", *Mitigation and Adaptation Strategies for Global Change*, Vol. 10, pp. 127–143, Springer

Kirksey, Eben and Stefan Helmreich 2010: The Emergence of Multispecies Ethnography, *Cultural Anthropology*, Vol. 25, Issue 4, pp. 54–576

Knorr-Cetina, Karin 1981: *The Manufacture of Knowledge: An Essay on the Constructivist and Contextual Nature of Science*. Pergamon Press: Oxford

Kohn, Eduardo 2007: How Dogs Dream: Amazonian Natures and the Politics of Transspecies Engagement. American Ethnologist Vol. 34, Issue 1, pp. –24

Kwa, Chunglin 2002: "Romantic and baroque conceptions of complex wholes in the sciences" pp. 23–52 in Law, John and Annemarie Mol (Eds.): *Complexities: Social Studies of Knowledge Practices*. Duke University Press, Durham, NC

Lakoff, Andrew and Stephen J. Collier (Eds.) 2008: *Biosecurity Interventions*, Columbia University *Press: New Yor*

*Latour, Bruno 1987: Science in Action: How to Follow Scientists and Engineers Through Society.* Milton Keynes: Open University Press

Latour, Bruno 1988: *The Pasteurization of France*. Cambridge, Massachusetts, Harvard

Latour, Bruno 1990: "Drawing things together", in Michael E. Lynch and Steve Woolgar (Eds.): R*epresentation in Scientific Practice*, MIT Press, Cambridge, Massachusett

Latour, Bruno 1999: *Pandora's Hope. Essays on the Reality of Science Studies*. Harward University Press, Cambridge, Massachusetts; London, England

Latour, Bruno 2004: "Why has critique run out of steam? From matters of fact to matters of concern", in *Critical Inquiry*, Vol. 30 pp. 22–24

Latour, Bruno 2005: "From Realpolitik to Dingpolitik or How to Make Things Public", pp. 14–41 in Bruno Latour and Peter Weibel (Eds.): *Making Things Public. Atmospheres of Democracy.* Cambridge, Massachusetts: The MIT Press

Latour, Bruno and Steve Woolgar 1979: *Laboratory Life: The Construction of Scientific Facts*. Sage Publications, Beverly Hills

Lavau, Stephanie 2008: *The Many Lives of the Goulburn River: Sustainable Management as Ontological Work.* Thesis Submitted in total fulfilment of the requirements of the degree of Doctor of Philosophy, School of Philosophy, Anthropology and Social Inquiry, The University of Melbourn

Law, John 1986: "On the methods of long distance control: vessels, navigation and the Portuguese route to India", in Law, John (Ed.): *Power, Action and*

*Belief: A New Sociology of Knowledge?* Sociological Review Monograph Vol. 32, pp. 234–263. Routledge and Kegan Paul, London.

Law, John 1994: *Organizing Modernity*, Blackwell Publishers, Oxford, UK

Law, John 2001: "Ordering and Obduracy", Centre for Science Studies, Lancaster University, Lancaster LA1 4YN, UK. (Revised. on 7th Dec. 2003)

Law, John 2002a: *Aircraft stories. Decentering the objects in technoscience.* Durham, North Carolina: Duke University Press

Law, John 2002b: "'On Hidden Heterogeneities: Complexity, Formalism and Aircraft Design', in John Law and Annemarie Mol (Eds): *Complexities: Social Studies of Knowledge Practices pages*, pp. 116–141. Durham, North Carolina: Duke University Press

Law, John 2003: "Making a Mess with Method," version of 19th January 2006. http://www.heterogeneities.net/publications/Law2006MakingaMesswithMethod.pdf, (downloaded on 17.11.2013)

Law, John 2004a: "And if the global were small and noncoherent? Method, complexity, and the baroque", *Environment and Planning D: Society and Space*, Vol. 22, pp. 13–26

Law, John 2004b: Matter-ing: or How Might STS Contribute? CSS, Lancaster University. (Revised on 3th June, 2004

Law, John 2011: "What is Wrong With a One-World World?", paper presented to the Center for the Humanities, Wesleyan University, Middletown, Connecticut on 19th September, http://www.heterogeneities.net/publications/Law2011WhatsWrongWithAOneWorldWorld.pdf, (accessed on 11.07.2014)

Law, John and John Hassard eds. 2006 [1999]:*Actor Network Theory and After*,Blackwell Publishers, Oxford, UK

Law, John and Annemarie Mol 2001: "Situating Technoscience: An Inquiry into Spatialities", *Society and Space*, Vol. 19, pp. 609–621

Law, John and Annemarie Mol 2008: "Globalisation in practice: On the politics of boiling pigswill", in *Geoforum* Vol. 39, pp. 13–14

Law, John and Ingunn Moser 2010: "Contexts and Culling", version of 16th March 2010, http://www.heterogeneities.net/publications/LawMoser2010ContextsCulling.pdf (downloaded on 30th March, 2010)

Leach, Melissa, Ian Scoones and Andrew Stirling 2010: *Governing epidemics in an age of complexity: Narratives, politics and pathways to sustainability*, Global Environmental Change Vol. 20, pp. 369–377

Lemke, Thomas 2014: "New Materialisms: Foucault and the 'Government of Things"',*Theory, Culture & Society*, Vol. 0 issue 0, pp. –23, Sage. Published online 2 April 2014 DOI: 10.1177/0263276413519340

Li, Tania Murray 2007:*The Will to Improve: Governmentality, Development, and the Practice of Politics.* Duke University Press Durham, NC

Lien, Marianne 2005: ",King of fish' or ,feral peril': Tasmanian Atlantic salmon and the politics of belonging" in*Environment and Planning D: Society and Space,* Vol. 23, Issue. 5, pp. 659–671

Liu, J., H. Xiao, F. Lei, Q. Zhu, K. Qin, X.-w. Zhang, X.-l. Zhang, D. Zhao, G. Wang, Y. Feng, J. Ma, W. Liu, J. Wang and G. F. Gao 2005: "Highly Pathogenic H5N1 Influenza Virus Infection in Migratory Birds", in*Science*, Vol. 309,19 AUGUST

Lowe, Celia 2010: "Viral Clouds: Becoming H5N1 in Indonesia", *Cultural Anthropology*, Vol. 25, Issue 4, pp. 62–64

Madsen, Linda 2004: *Technical Solutions to Industrial Pollution. The Case of Textile Industry in Turkey*. Unpublished Master Thesis, Faculty of Social Sciences, University of Oslo

MARA 2001: *Instruction on Protection from and Fight Against Avian Influenza.* The republic of Turkey Ministry of Agriculture and Rural Affairs, General Directorate of Protection and Control. Ankar

MARA 2005: *Report on Avian Influenza in Turkey*, Ministry of Agriculture, General Directorate for Protection and Control, http://www.kkgm.gov.tr/birim/hay_sagl/Hastaliklar/AI/AI_WEB/2005_bildirim/ABraporlari-2005/21.12.2005.pdf, downloaded on 18.04.2011

MARA 2006*: Preparation of Sector Analyses for Certain Agricultural Products: Poultry Meat Sector*. Agri-Livestock Consultants Ltd. November. Ministry of Agriculture and Rural Affairs. Turke

MARA/KKGM 2008 Sazkoy: A*vian Influenza in Zonguldak – State of Play. 25.01.2008 Zonguldak-Caycuma-Sazkoy.* Report from the Republic of Turkey Ministry of Agriculture and Rural Affairs. Ankara

Marcus, George 1995: "Ethnography in/of the World System: The Emergence of Multi-Sited Ethnography", in *Annual Review of Anthropology*, Vol. 24, pp. 95–117

Marcus, George and Judith Okley 2008: "How short can fieldwork be?" debate in *Social Anthropology/Anthropologie Sociale*, Vol. 15,Issue 3, pp. 1–15

Massey, Doreen 1995:*Spatial Division of Labour: Social Structures and the Geography of Production*. Macmillan: Londo

Massey, Doreen 2004: "Geographies of responsibility." *Geografiska Annaler: Series B, Human Geography*, Vol. 86, Issue 1, pp. –18

Massey, Doreen 2009 [2005]:*For space*, Sage: Los Angeles, London, New Deli, Singapore, Washington DC

Matthews, Christopher 2006: *Free as a bird – or under surveillance? Plan for global wild bird tracking system*, FAO Newsroom. As of 20.08.2014 available on: http://www.fao.org/newsroom/en/news/2006/1000311/index.html

Mol, Annemarie 1998: “Lived reality and the multiplicity of norms: a critical tribute to George Canguilhem”, in *Econmy and Society*, Vol. 27, pp. 274–28

Mol, Annemarie 2002: *The Body Multiple: Ontology in medical practise*. Duke University Press

Mol, Annemarie 2005 [1999]: “Ontological Politics: a Word and Some Questions”, pp. 74–89 in John Law and John Hassard (Eds): *Actor Network Theory and After*, Oxford and Keele: Blackwell and the Sociological Review

Mol, Annemarie and Law John 1994: “Regions, networks and fluids: anaemia and social topology” in *Social Studies of Science,* Vol. 24, pp. 641–671

Moreira, Tiago 2009: “Testing promises: Truth and hope in drug development and evaluation in Alzheimer’s disease”, in Jesse F. Ballenger, Peter J. Whitehouse, Constantine Lyketsos, Peter Rabins & Jason H. T. Karlawish (Eds.): *Treating dementia. Do we have a pill for that?*, Baltimore: Johns Hopkins University Press

Morse, Stephen S. ed. 1993: *Emerging viruses*, Oxford University Press. Oxford

Moser, Ingunn Brita 2003: *Road Traffic Accidents: The ordering of Subjects, Bodies and Disability*. Doctoral Dissertation, Faculty of Arts, University of Oslo, Unipub AS, Oslo

Moser, Ingunn 2005: “On Becoming Disabled and Articulating Alternatives”, in *Cultural Studie*s Vol. 19, Issue. 6, pp. 667–70

Moser; Ingunn 2008: “Making Alzheimer’s disease matter. Enacting, interfering and doing politics of nature”, *Geoforum* Vol. 39 pp. 98–110. Elsevier

Moser, Ingunn 2011: ”Normalitetens grenser, pris og alternativer – funksjonshemning som levd realitet.” Kronikk i *Tidsskrift for den Norske Laegeforening*, Vol. 131, Issue 9, 962.

Mylius, Christian Otto, (Ed.) 1740, *Corpus Constitutionum Marchicarum*. Berlin, 5: Part 4,423–424 (No. 1), Patent of 14 September 166; 5: Part 4, 42–425 (No. 2), Patent of 1667 and 5: Part 4, 425428 (No. 3), Patent of 1682.

Nerlich, Brigitte and Nick Wright 2006: “Biosecurity and Insecurity: The Interaction between Policy and Ritual During the Foot and Mouth Crisis”,*Environmental Value*s, Vol. 15, pp. 44–62

Newman, Scott, Nick Honhold, Javier Sanz-Alvarez and Kiraz Erciyas 2008: *Investigation of the role of wild birds in highly pathogenic avian influenza outbreaks in Turkey between January and February 2008*. Mission Report, Food and Agriculture Organization of the United Nations, Crisis Management Centre – Animal Health and Animal Health Division- EMPRES, Rome, Italy. As of 20.08.2014 available on: http://www.fao.org/docs/eims/upload//263862/ak142e00.pdf

NFU in BBC 2007: BBC, 2007 Farming Today This Week, Radio 4, 11 August

Normille, Dennis 2005: "Avian influenza: Are Wild Birds to Blame?" *Science* October 21th, Vol. 310, no. 5747, pp. 426–428

Nævestad, Tor-Olav 2009: "Mapping Research on Culture and Safety in High-Risk Organizations: Arguments for a Sociotechnical Understanding of Safety Culture", in *Journal of Contingencies and Crisis Management*, Vol. 17, Issue 2, pp. 126–136,

OIE 2008/3: *Bulletin*, No. 2008, Issue 3, World Organization for Animal Health. Paris

Okumus, Kerem (Ed.) 2002: *Turkey's Environment.A Review and Evaluation of Turkey's Environment and its Stakeholders*. The Regional Environmental Center for Central and Eastern Europe. Szentendre, Hungary

Ong, Aihwa 1999: *Flexible Citizenship. The Cultural Logics of Trans nationality.* Duke University Press

Ong, Aihwa and Stephen J. Collier (Eds.) 2005: *Global Assemblages. Technology, Politics, and Ethics as Anthropological Problems.* Wiley

Oudshoorn, Nelly 1999: "The Decline of the One-Size-Fits-All Approach. Or: How Reproductive Scienctists Try to Cope with Postmodernity" pp. 153–173 in R. Braidotti and N. Lykke: *Between Monsters, Goddesses and Cyborgs: Feminist Confrontations with Science, Medicine, and Cyberspace*, ZED Books, London

Perrow, Charles 1999: *Normal Accidents: Living With High Risk Technologies*, Princeton

Porter, Natalie 2013a: "Bird flu biopower: Strategies for multispecies coexistence in Viet Nam",*American Ethnologis*t, Vol. 40, No. 1, pp. 132–148, ISSN 0094–049

Porter, Natalie 2013b: "Global Health Cadres: Avian Flu Control and Practical Statecraft in Vietnam", in*Journal of Social Issues in Southeast Asia*, Volume 28, Number 1, March 2013, pp. 64–100, Institute of Southeast Asian Studies

Porter, Natalie 2014 forthcoming: "Bird flu counter conduct in Vietnam", in Kristin Asdal, Marianne Lien, Steve Hinchliffe and Tone Druglitrø (Eds.): *Sentient creatures: transforming biopolitics and life matters.* London: Ashgate

Rabinow, Paul and Nikolas Rose 2006: "Biopower today", *BioSocieties* 1, pp. 195–217

Roe; Emery and Paul R. Schulman 2008: *High Reliability Management: Operating at the Edge*, Stanford University Press, Palo Alto

Rose, Nikolas 1999: *Powers of Freedom. Reframing Political Thought*, Cambridge

Rosenberg, Charles E. 1992: *Explaining Epidemics: and Other Studies in the History of Medicine*. Cambridge: Cambridge University Press

Sariözkan Savaş, Cengiz Yalcin, Yavu Cevger, YilmazAral and Ceva Sipahi 2009: "The Financial Impacts Of The Avian Influenza Outbreaks On Turkish Table Egg Producers", *Worlds Poultry Science Journal*, Vol. 65, Issue 1, pp. 91–96

Sauer, Carl Ortwin [1925], 1963: "The morphology of landscape" in J. Leighley, (Ed.): *Land and life: selections from the writings of Carl Ortwin Sauer*, University of California Press: Berkeley

Sayed H. Saghaian, Gökhan Özertan, and Aslıhan D. Spaulding 2008: "Dynamics of Price Transmission in the Presence of a Major Food Safety Shock: Impact of H5N1 Avian Influenza on the Turkish Poultry Sector," in*Journalof Agricultural and Applied Economics*, Vol. 40, Issue 3, pp. 1015–1031

Scoones, Ian (Ed.) 2010: *Avian Influenza. Science, Policy and Politics.* Earthscan: London, Washington DC

Scoones, Ian and Paul Forster 2008: "The International Response to Highly Pathogenic Avian Influenza: Science, Policy and Politics", *STEPS Working Paper 10*, STEPS Centre: Brighton http://steps-centre.org/wp-content/uploads/STEPS-_Working-Paper_Avian-Flu.pdf, (*accessed on 15.07.2014*)

Scott, Gordon R. and Alain Provost 1992: *Global Eradication of Rinderpest,* FAO-Food and Agricultural Organization of the United Nations: Edinburgh

Serres, Michel 1995: *Conversations on Science, Culture, and Time: Michel Serres with Bruno Latour.* Studies in Literature and Science. University of Michigan Press: United States of America

Sevindik, Durmuş, Seçkin Kirarslan, Ünal Uzun 2008: "Saz Köyü'nde kuş gribi karantinası", Milliyet 22.02.2008. As of 20.08.2014 available on: http://www.milliyet.com.tr/2008/01/22/son/sontur44.asp

Shapin, Steven and Simon Schaffer 1985: *Leviathan and the Air-Pump: Hobbes, Boyle, and the Experimental Life*. Princeton University Press, Princeton, New Jersey

Singleton, Vicky 2005: "The promise of public health: vulnerable policy and lazy citizens" i*Environment and Planning D: Society and Space*, Vol. 23, pp. 771–786

Singleton, Vicky 2010: "Good farming. Control are Care?" in care in Annemarie Mol, Ingunn Moser and Jeannette Pols (Eds.): *Care in Practise. On Thinkering in Clinics, Homes and Farms*. transcript Verlag, Bielefeld

Sipahi, Ceva, Cengiz. Yalcin, Yavu Cevger, YilmazAral and L. Genc 2011: "Small-Scale Family Poultry Production Impact of avian influenza outbreaks on Turkish village chicken producers, and their opinions on the disease and disease control", in World's Poultry Science Journal Vol. 67, Issue 1, pp. 131–136

Star, Susan Leigh 1991: "Power Technology and the Phenomenology of Conventions. On Being Allergic to Onions", in John Law (Ed.): *A Sociology of Monsters. Essays on Power, Technology and Domination*. Sociological Review Monograph Vol. 38. Reprinted in Asdal, Kristin, Brita Brenna and Ingunn Moser 2007: *Technoscience. The Politics of Interventions*, Unipub

Stirling, Andy S. and Ian Scoones 2009: "From Risk Assessment to Knowledge Mapping: Science, Precaution, and Participation in Disease Ecology", in*Ecology and Society*, Vol. 14, Issue 2 http://www.ecologyandsociety.org/vol14/iss2/art14/ecologyandsociety.org/vol14/iss2/art14/, (downloaded on 15.07.2014)

Strathern, Marilyn 2004 [1991]: *Partial connections*. Savage, Md.: Rowman and Littlefield

Sundqvist, Göran and Mark Elam 2010: "Public Involvement Designed to Circumvent Public Concern? The 'Participatory Turn' in European Nuclear Activities", in*Risk, Hazards & Crisis in Public Policy*, Vol. 1, Issus 4, Art. 8, pp. 203–229

Sur, Haydar et.al 2007: *Turkey Avian Influenza Knowledge, Attitude, Practices, Behavior Research*, Report carried out by Marmara University Health Training Faculty, financed by UNICEF

Swayne, D. E. and D. L. Suarez 2000: "Highly pathogenic avian influenza", inBeard, C.W. and M.S. McNulty (Eds.) 2000: *Diseases of poultry: world trade and public health implications*. World Organisation for Animal Health Scientific and Technical Review Issue 19, Vol. 2, pp. 463–482. http://www.oie.int/doc/ged/D9311.PDF, (accessed on*26.01.2014*)

Tokuş, Zaferm, Arife Balta, Aziz Güvner 2008: "Sakarya'da kuş gribi", in *Hürriyet* [newspaper] online 05.02.2008 http://www.hurriyet.com.tr/gundem/8171620.asp?m=1, (accessed on 04.08.2014)

Traweek Sharon 1992: *Beamtimes and Lifetimes: The World of High Energy Physicists*, Harward University Press, United States of America

Tsing, Anna L. 2005: *Friction: An Ethnography of Global Connection*, Princeton University Press

Tsuda, Takeyuki, Maria Tapias and Xavier Escandell 2014: "Locating the Global in Transnational Ethnography", in *Journal of Contemporary Ethnography*, Vol. 43, Issue 2, pp. 123–14

UNEP/CMS 2007: Proceedings of the 2nd Technical Meeting of the Scientific Task Force on Avian Influenza & Wild Birds, Avian Influenza & Wildlife Workshop on 'Practical Lessons Learned, Aviemore, Scotland: 26 – 28 June

Vallat, Bernard 2011: "The Odyssey of Rinderpest Eradication". Editorial, OIE – World organization for Animal Health, http://www.oie.int/for-the-media/editorials/detail/article/the-odyssey-of-rinderpest-eradication/, (accessed on 27.04.2014)

Van den Ende, Marinus and Ragip Bayraktar 2008 Esetce: *Avian Influenza Outbreak Mission Report in Esetce village / Ipsala District / Edirne Province*, pp. 53 – 74. Technical Assistance to Avian Influenza Preparedness and Response Project, Turkey. As of 21.08.2014 avaiable on: http://www.prwatson.co.uk/TR_06_AI_SV/English/Reports/AI %20outbreak%20mission%20reports.pdf

Van den Ende, Rinus and Ragip Bayraktar 2008 Sazkoy: *Avian Influenza Outbreak Investigation Mission Report in Sazkoy Village / Zonguldak province 22–23 January 2008.* Technical Assistance to Avian Influenza Preparedness and Response Project, Turkey. As of 21.08.2014 avaiable on: http://www.prwatson.co.uk/TR_06_AI_SV/English/Reports/ Sazkoy%20oubreak.pdf

Weber, Thomas P. and Nikolaos I. Stilianakis 2007: "Ecologic Immunology of Avian Influenza (H5N1) in Migratory Birds", in*Emerging Infectious Diseases* Vol. 13, No. 8, August 2007

Whatmore, Sarah 2006: "Materialist Returns: Practicing Cultural Geography in and for a More-Than-Human World", Author manuscript, published in *Cultural Geographies* Vol. 13, issue 4, pp. 600–609

WHO 2005: *Responding to the Avian Influenza Pandemic Threat*, WHO/CDS/CSR/GIP/2005.8. http://www.who.int/csr/resources/publications/influenza/WHO_CDS_CSR_GIP_05_8-EN.pdf, (accessed on 14.03.2014)

WHO 2006: *Making preparation count: lessons from the avian influenza outbreak inTurkey*. Report, World Health Organization. ISBN 92–890–1386–9, http://www.euro.who.int/__data/assets/pdf_file/0018/90513/E89139.pdf, (accessed on 09.05.2014)

Wright, Susan 1986: "Molecular Biology or Molecular Politics? The Production of Scientific Consensus on the Hazards of Recombinant DNA Technology", in *Social Studies of Science*, Vol. 16, pp. 593–620(SAGE. London. Beverly Hills and New Delhi

Wolf, Meike 2012: Influenza and the Concept of Infection: Reflections on Bodily Boundaries" in *Antropologij*a Vol. 12, Issue. 2, pp. 107–121

Wulff Helena 2002: "Yo-Yo Fieldwork: Mobility and Time in a Multilocal Study of Dance in Ireland" in *Anthropological Journal of European Cultures. Shifting Grounds – Experiments in Doing Ethnography,* Vol. 117–136

Yalcin, Cengiz 2006: *Market Impacts of HPAI Outbreaks: A Rapid Appraisal Process– Turke*y. Paper presented at Symposium on The Market and Trade Dimensions of Avian Influenza, Rome, Italy, 14 November 2006, report submitted to FAO and online available http://www.fao.org/docs/eims/upload/234380/ah675e00.pdf, (accessed on 11.07.2014)

Yalcin, Cengiz, Cevat Sipahi, Yilmaz Aral, and Yavuz Cevger 2010: "Economic Effect of the Highly Pathogenic Avian Influenza H5N1 Outbreaks Among Turkey Producers, 200–06, Turkey," in *Avian Diseases*, Vol. 54, Issue, pp. 39–393

## Websites and pages:

AI project/Technical Assistance to Avian Influenza Preparedness and Response Project web site, available as of 21.08.2014 on: http://www.prwatson.co.uk/TR_06_AI_SV/English/start.htm, (*accessed on 18.07.2014*)

European Commission, Enlargement Detailed information on Turkey. As of 20.08.2014 available on: http://ec.europa.eu/enlargement/countries/detailed-country-information/turkey/index_en.htm, (*accessed on 05.03.2013*)

FAO Biosecurity for Agriculture and Food Production, website. As of 20.08.2014 available on: http://www.fao.org/biosecurity/, italics in original, (*accessed on 16.07.2014*)

OIE on Emerging and re-emerging zoonoses. As of 20.08.2014 available on: http://www.oie.int/for-the-media/editorials/detail/article/emerging-and-re-emerging-zoonoses/

OIE 2011: "Post Eradication Phase" webpage on site *2011: Global Rinderpest eradication.* http://www.oie.int/for-the-media/rinderpest/,(*accessed on 16.07.2014*)

OIE (GF-TADs): The Global Framework for the Progressive Control of Transboundary Animal Diseases (GF-TADs), Version approved as basic text the

24 May 2004 by FAO and OIE) http://www.oie.int/rr-europe/eng/Projects /GF-TADs_2004.pdf, *accessed on 10.01.2014*

OIE/ Terrestrial Codex, Chapter 10.4 Avian influenza Art.10.4.1, http://web.oie.int/eng/normes/mcode/en_chapitre_1.10.4.pdf, (*accessed on 09.05.2014*)

OIE /Wahid, Immediate notification report received 07.10.2005 from Mr Gabriel Predoi, Direction générale sanitaire vétérinaire, Directeur général, Bucarest,Romania. http://www.oie.int/wahis_2/public/wahid.php/Review report/Review?reportid=5189, (*accessed on 26.03.2014*)

OIE /Wahid, Immediate Notification Report, reference: Ref OIE: 5306, Report Date: 10/10/2005, Country: Turkey, http://web.oie.int/wahis/reports/en_imm_0000005306_20051010_172322.pdf, (*accessed on 16.07.2014*)

OIE /Wahid, Follow-up Report No 2, date of report 14.10.2005 http://www.oie.int/wahis_2/public/wahid.php/Reviewreport/Review?reportid=5204, (*accessed on 26.03.2014*)

Ramsar Convention on Wetlands website. *As of 20.08.2014 accessed on*: http://www.ramsar.org/cda/en/ramsar-home/main/ramsar/1_4000_0__,

United Nations Avian Influenza and the Pandemic Threat website. *As of 20.08.2014 accessed on: http://un-influenza.org, accessed on 27.11.2013*

U.S. Central Intelligence Agency 2006: *Turkey (Political) [Map] 2006*, University of Texas Libraries, http://www.ecoi.net/file_upload/470_1284541589_turkey-pol-2006.jpg, (*accessed on* 11.08.2014)

WHO on Emerging Diseases. *As of 20.08.2014 accessed on*: http://www.who.int/topics/emerging_diseases/en

## Field notes and interviews cited:

15.05.2007: Personal communication with Director of Finances, Poultry Producing Company, Balıkeşir.

Field notes: 15.05.2007 Kızıksa village, Manyas District, Balıkesir Province.

29.05.2007: Interview with international field epidemiologist working for the AI project, Ankara.

11. and 12.06.2007: Personal communication with two recovered avian influenza victims, Van.

11.06.2007: Personal communication/interview with Prof. Dr. Ahment Faik Üner, Van University Hospital.

16.06.2007: Personal communication with veterinary working for Ağrı Provincial Directorate of Agriculture and Rural Affairs, Ağrı.

31.01.2008: Personal communication with epidemiological expert, Ankara.

15.10.2008: Field notes Esetçe village, Ipsala District, Edirne Province.
21.10.2008: Field notes Konacık village, Karasu District, Sakarya Province.
24.10.2008: Field notes Kaynarca/Sakarya.